THE ESSENTIAL MASSAGE BOOK

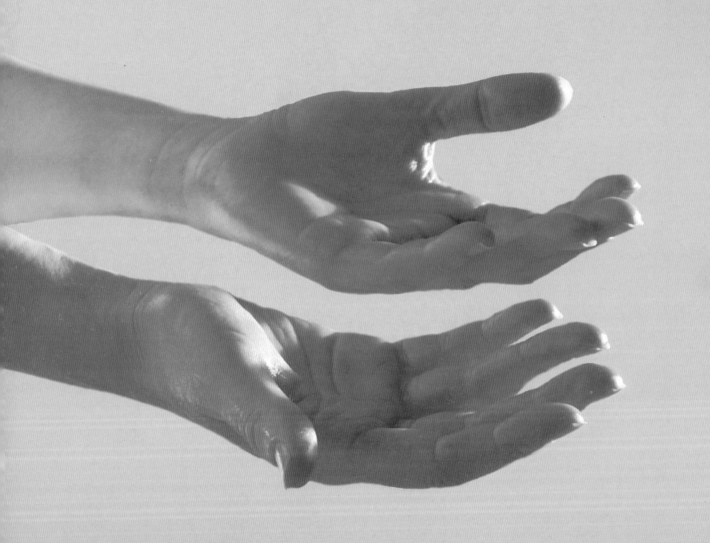

THE ESSENTIAL MASSAGE BOOK

GENERAL EDITOR
Eilean Bentley

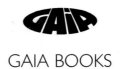

GAIA BOOKS

A GAIA ORIGINAL

Books from Gaia celebrate the vision of Gaia, the self-sustaining
living Earth, and seek to help its readers live in greater personal
and planetary harmony.

Editors Katherine Pate, Kelly Thompson
Designer Bridget Morley
Photography Sam Scott-Hunter, Fausto Dorelli
Production Simone Nauerth
Direction Jo Godfrey Wood, Patrick Nugent

First published in the United Kingdom in 2005 by
Gaia Books, an imprint of
Octopus Publishing Group, 2-4 Heron Quays, London E14 4JP

ISBN 1 85675 203 8
EAN 9 781856 752039

615.822

A catalogue record of this book is available from the British Library.

Printed and bound in China by Toppan

10 9 8 7 6 5 4 3 2 1

CAUTIONS AND CONTRAINDICATIONS

All the massage treatments recommended in this book are extremely safe. However, there are certain conditions and illnesses for which massage is not recommended. Cautions relating to specific steps of a massage are explained in the step-by-step treatments. Please also observe the cautions listed below. At all times, if you are unsure whether massage is appropriate, first check with a doctor.

Do not massage directly over broken, inflamed, or infectious skin conditions, bruises, varicose veins, recent scar tissue, tumours or any undiagnosed lumps, or cardiovascular problems such as thrombosis or phlebitis. Gentle work on unaffected areas of the body can be very soothing and comforting. Do not massage during high fever.

Use only light massage on the very young, the very old, and anyone with bone problems. Pressure should not exceed the weight of your fingers; even the weight of your hand can be excessive, especially on the top of the head.

People undergoing conventional treatment for cancer should consult their doctor before having any massage treatment. Gentle massage can be of great benefit, but avoid working on the lymphatic areas on the side of the face, the throat, across the chin, and behind the ears, since lymph can transport some forms of cancer cells around the body.

In some cases, massage can bring about an emotional release, which may manifest in tears or flu-like symptoms for a few days afterward.

Shiatsu

Do not give shiatsu on the abdomen of anyone who is pregnant, and do not use strong pressure on the tops of the shoulders. During the later stages of pregnancy, avoid heavy pressure on the legs. For people with high blood pressure or epilepsy, do not give shiatsu on the top of the head; work on the limbs, especially the legs and feet, is beneficial and safe. Avoid leaning heavily on elderly or infirm people, especially those with brittle bones.

Chinese massage

Some acupoints should not be treated in particular circumstances. These points are clearly indicated in the step-by-step massage treatments. In particular, do not treat the following points on anyone who is pregnant: Sp6, LI4, GB21, Ren3, Ren4, GB26, St29, St36, Sp12, and B60.

Aromatherapy massage

For people who have high blood pressure, epilepsy, or a progressive neural disorder, the actions of some essential oils may adversely affect their condition. Before using essential oils, consult a professional aromatherapist or medical herbalist.

Reiki

Do not use: on people with mental health problems, including depression; on people with a pacemaker or other electrically stimulated implant; over broken bones until medical treatment has been given; on anyone who is under anaesthetic, as it may counteract the anaesthetic's effect. These cautions also apply to distance healing.

Only use hands-off techniques over broken, inflamed, or infectious skin conditions.

Head massage

Head massage lowers the blood pressure, so anyone who already has low blood pressure should only have a light treatment, lasting no longer than 15 minutes. The top of the head is a particularly sensitive area for people with epilepsy or clinical depression. Use light massage only, no more than stroking or combing with your fingers.

Reflexology

Always seek advice from a professional reflexologist before treating women during the first 14 weeks of pregnancy, and people with diabetes, thrombosis, or phlebitis.

CONTENTS

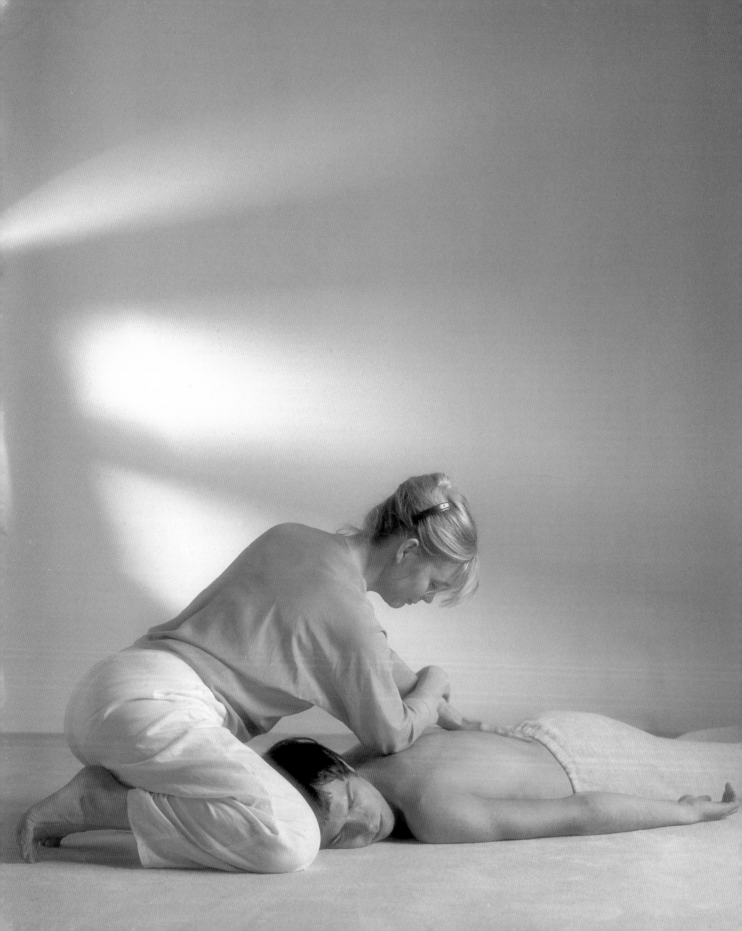

HOW TO USE THIS BOOK

The Essential Book of Massage presents illustrated step-by-step instructions for massage treatments from a wide range of traditions: holistic massage, Chinese massage, shiatsu, Reiki, intuitive massage, aromatherapy, reflexology, and head massage.

Chapter 1, Introduction to massage, explains the theory behind each type of massage, and how to perform the basic strokes used in the treatments in later chapters. The final section of this chapter gives advice on preparing yourself and the room before you give a massage, and how to begin and end a treatment session.

The sequences in chapters 2 to 7 take you through massage treatments for the whole body. The next two chapters focus on massaging specific areas: reflexology on the feet in chapter 8 and head massage in chapter 9. Chapter 10 presents short self-massage sequences, and chapter 11 highlights techniques from a variety of massage styles that promote relaxation. The Tantric sexual massage sequence in chapter 12 creates deeper intimacy between lovers.

You may like to begin by reading chapter 1 and deciding which style of massage you feel drawn to try first. Alternatively, you may have already decided which massage treatment to try. In either case, practising the basic strokes for that form of massage, described in chapter 1, will make it easier to follow the step-by-step instructions in the massage treatment.

The charts in the Appendix are useful reference for the different massage sequences. They include the Channels and acupoints used in Chinese massage and shiatsu, reflexology maps of the feet and hands, the qualities of essential oils for aromatherapy, and the location and qualities of the Chakras for Reiki and Tantra. The body landmarks chart on page 252 illustrates the major bones and muscles, to help you locate areas to treat.

Massage can provide us with a means to counteract the relentless surge of work and domestic pressures. For all too many of us, stiffness and pain are a way of life to which we have become habituated, and often it is not until we give or receive massage that we realize that our muscles are tight, or how much of our energy is consumed by tension. Massage can be a voyage of self-discovery, revealing how it feels to be more relaxed and in tune with ourselves, to experience the pleasure of a body that can breathe, stand, and move freely.

INTRODUCTION TO MASSAGE

For thousands of years, some form of massage or laying on of hands has been used to heal and soothe the sick. In the East, massage techniques have been valued for their healing applications and used since earliest times. The instinctive desire to "rub it better", combined with skills refined and elaborated by long tradition and Oriental medical theory, gave rise to Traditional Chinese Massage, and shiatsu in Japan.

To the ancient Greek and Roman physicians, massage was one of the principal means of relieving pain. Early in the 5th century BC, Hippocrates – the "father of medicine" – wrote: "The physician must be experienced in many things, but assuredly in rubbing ... For rubbing can bind a joint that is too loose, and loosen a joint that is too rigid." Pliny, the renowned Roman naturalist, was regularly "rubbed" to relieve his asthma and Julius Caesar, who suffered from epilepsy, was daily pinched all over to ease his neuralgia and headaches.

After the fall of Rome in the 5th century AD, the Europeans made little progress in the medical sphere and it was left to the Arabs to study and develop the teachings of the classical world. Avicenna, the 11th century Arab philosopher and physician, noted in his Canon that the object of massage was "to disperse the effete matters found in the muscles and not expelled by exercise".

During the Middle Ages, little was heard of massage in Europe, due to the contempt for pleasures of the flesh. But it was revived in the 16th century, mainly through the work of a French doctor, Ambroise Paré. Then, at the beginning of the 19th century, a Swede by the name of Per Henrik Ling developed what is now known as Swedish massage, synthesizing his system from his knowledge of gymnastics and physiology and from Chinese, Egyptian, Greek, and Roman techniques. Today the therapeutic value of massage has once more been recognized and it continues to flourish and develop throughout the Western world, both among lay practitioners and professionals.

The following pages outline the theory behind the types of massage used in this book, and the basic strokes and techniques you will need for the sequences described in chapters 2 to 12.

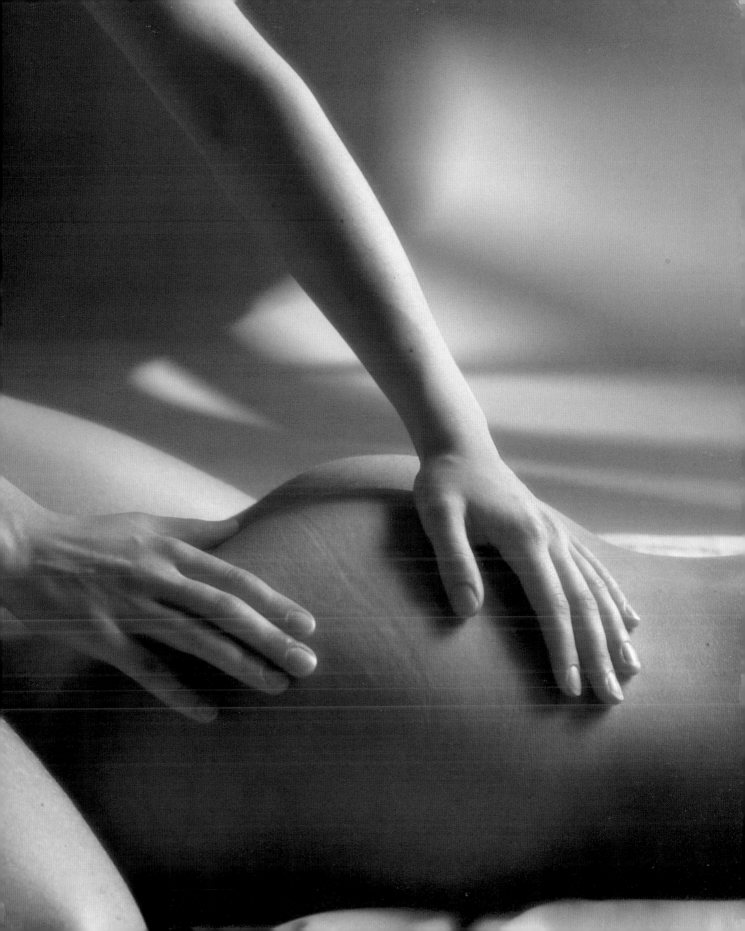

HOLISTIC MASSAGE

Massage is the sharing of touch, yet it goes further than skin deep, deeper even than muscles or bones – a good, caring massage penetrates right to the depth of your being.

Physically, its benefits include relaxing and toning the muscles; assisting the venous flow of blood; soothing the nervous system; encouraging lymphatic flow; and stretching the connective tissue of joints. Holistic massage also affects the Chakras. On a mental level, it relieves stress and anxiety and also helps you to become more conscious of your body as a whole, of the parts that you are in touch with and of those that feel "cut off". Once you are aware of where your energy blocks lie, you can begin to integrate your body and, in developing a more positive self-image, take responsibility for your own happiness and health.

Holistic massage treats the individual as a whole, and its movements are generally slow, rhythmic, and meditative. Throughout the massage, the giver should try to remain "centred", transmitting caring love to the receiver.

BASIC STROKES

The basic strokes used in holistic massage are presented here. You can practise these before giving the holistic massage whole-body treatment (pages 32–67) or using the self-massage sequence (pages 198–9). Other techniques used are described in the step-by-step instructions for those sequences.

To the receiver, the massage should feel like one continuous sequence, in which the strokes flow rhythmically from one into the other. Remember that any tension or awkwardness in your posture will be felt by your partner. If you practise letting your whole body move from the hips, rather than using just your arms and hands, you will find that your hands relax and the strokes come naturally to you.

The Chakras

According to Eastern mystical tradition, every person has seven Chakras – centres of energy in the etheric body – which spin like wheels, enabling pure life force to be absorbed. Each Chakra has a particular energy frequency and relates to the organs in the body that resonate with that frequency. These organs absorb and distil this energy, and then radiate it out as a particular quality. The Chakras, with their related organs and qualities, are shown on page 251.

Thumb rolling

Press the pads of your thumbs firmly into your partner's flesh, using short, deep strokes or small circles, depending on where you are working. Bring one thumb down just behind the other, but push on a little further with each successive stroke so that you eventually cover a fairly broad area. This technique works deep into the tissues to release hidden tensions.

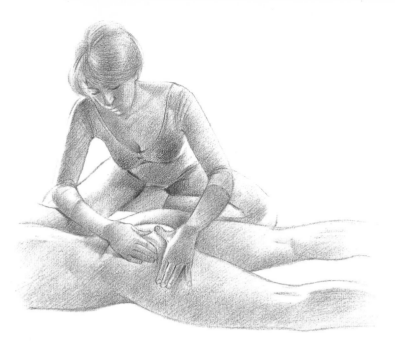

Kneading

Using your whole hands, alternately grasp and squeeze bunches of flesh – one hand releasing its hold as the other starts to gather a new handful. Don't lift the hands off the body between strokes; rock smoothly from hand to hand as if you were kneading dough. This technique stretches and releases soft, fleshy areas, such as buttocks and thighs.

Wringing

Place your left hand on your partner's nearest side, heel down, and your right hand on the far side, fingers down. Now push firmly forward with your left hand, and pull back with your right (A). Without stopping, change direction and wring the hands back to the opposite side (B). Move slowly along with each new stroke, keeping the flow continuous. This technique works on large muscle masses.

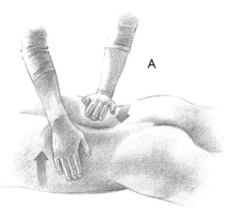

Gliding

Like waves rippling over rocks, these gentle rhythmic strokes glide over the skin. They are used on all parts of the body to begin and end a massage, and as transitional strokes to flow from one movement to another. They are also used to spread oil evenly over the body.

Keep your hands relaxed so that their whole surface comes into contact with your partner's body. Start by letting your hands float down to rest for a few seconds on the receiver. Then move both hands together slowly along the torso or limb, moulding them to the curves of the body. When you come to the end of your reach, separate your hands and glide them back up the sides, circling to return to the starting position.

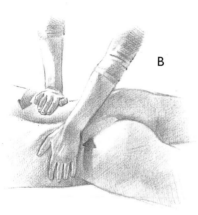

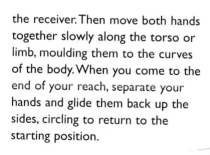

CHINESE MASSAGE

Chinese massage, along with acupuncture and herbalism, is part of the system of Traditional Chinese Medicine (TCM) used in China for over 2000 years. It is a natural and physical therapy that follows the fundamental rule of Chinese medicine: "To cure disease you must cure its root". To understand how Chinese massage promotes health and wellbeing, you first need an understanding of the basic concepts of Chinese medicine.

YIN AND YANG

TCM offers us a unique and exclusive answer to the age-old questions "What is life?" and "How is life created?" It tells us that the basis of all life is the interaction of Yin and Yang.

Yin and Yang are the opposite aspects of matter and phenomena in nature, and are both complementary and interdependent. Everything in the universe has Yin and Yang characteristics, and similarly all elements of the human body can be viewed as either more Yin or more Yang. When you are in full health, these two aspects are in perfect balance.

QI AND BLOOD

These are the two essential substances needed to support life. Qi can be thought of as the vital energy or life force – the primary motive force for all activities of life. Its two fundamental functions are to nourish the body and to protect it from external damage. Qi and blood support and complement each other: blood needs Qi to keep it moving and Qi is generated by blood.

Qi and blood circulate through energetic pathways called Channels or Meridians (see page 15) as "Qi–blood flow". In healthy conditions, Qi–blood flows smoothly. However, if the flow is disturbed Qi–blood stagnates, causing ill health or disease. The aim of Chinese massage is to influence Qi–blood flow to ensure it is smooth and regular.

THE ORGANS

The term "Organ" has a wider meaning in Chinese medicine than in Western thinking. For example, in Chinese medicine the Kidney is responsible not only for water metabolism but also for providing a link between sources of energy and growth, the bones and brain. In this book, we distinguish the Chinese concept of an organ by giving it an initial capital letter.

There are twelve principal Organs, known as the Zang–Fu. The Zang Organs, which are Yin, are the Lung, Pericardium, Heart, Spleen, Liver, and Kidney. The Fu Organs, which are Yang, are the Large Intestine, Triple Warmer, Small Intestine, Stomach, Gall Bladder, and Bladder.

THE CHANNEL SYSTEM

A system of Channels (or Meridians) – energy pathways through which Qi and blood flow – was precisely described in the first Chinese medical book, *Nei Jing*, more than 2000 years ago. The system consists of twelve Regular Channels, eight Extra

The Pericardium and Triple Warmer have no equivalent in Western medicine. The Pericardium protects and assists the Heart. The Triple Warmer regulates the flow of Qi and body fluids through the abdomen.

Causes of Qi–blood stagnation

According to TCM, there are Six Evils or external factors that can upset Qi–blood flow: Wind, Cold, Summer-heat, Damp, Dryness, and Fire. Normally our bodies can adapt to small changes in these factors, but if one or more are in excess or in short supply, Qi disturbance and stagnation may occur.

Stagnation can also result from internal pathogenic factors, such as an irregular lifestyle, exhaustion, and excess of the Seven Extreme Emotions: over-excitement, anxiety, anger, worry, grief, fear, and shock.

THE EXTERIOR–INTERIOR RELATIONSHIP BETWEEN THE YIN AND YANG CHANNELS

INTERIOR

LUNG CHANNEL

SPLEEN CHANNEL

HEART CHANNEL

KIDNEY CHANNEL

PERICARDIUM CHANNEL

LIVER CHANNEL

YIN

EXTERIOR

LARGE INTESTINE CHANNEL

STOMACH CHANNEL

SMALL INTESTINE CHANNEL

BLADDER CHANNEL

TRIPLE WARMER CHANNEL

GALL BLADDER CHANNEL

YANG

Channels, and some collaterals. The Chinese massage sequences in this book work on the twelve Regular Channels and two of the Extra Channels – Ren and Du. These Channels are illustrated on pages 240–41.

The Regular Channels are distributed symmetrically on both sides of the body and form six pairs. One Channel in each pair is Yin, the other Yang, forming an exterior–interior relationship. Generally the Yin Channels flow upward on the inside surfaces of the front of the body, and the Yang Channels flow downward on the outer surfaces on the back, with each Channel joining its pair at the end of a limb. Each Regular Channel also connects with an Organ, after which it is named, for example the Bladder Channel, or Lung Channel.

The two Extra Channels, the Ren and Du, are on the midline of the body.

ACUPOINTS
The Chinese word for "acupoint" means "small hole for Qi". The hundreds of acupoints along the course of the Channels help to transmit Qi and blood through the Channels. In addition, there are also Extraordinary acupoints, which are not on the Channels. Massaging the acupoints regulates Qi–blood flow to disperse stagnation and promote good health and wellbeing.

The acupoints on the Channels are identified by the name of the Channel and a number, for example Bladder 23 (abbreviated to B23). Extraordinary acupoints are known by their Chinese names, for example "Yintang". All the acupoints used in the sequences in this book are shown in the charts on pages 242–5 in the Appendix, with detailed instructions to help you locate them.

BASIC STROKES

These two pages show the basic techniques used in Chinese massage. Familiarize yourself with these before giving the Chinese massage whole-body treatment (pages 68–91) or using the self-massage treatment (pages 200–203).

Pressing

Use your finger, knuckle, or thumb to press an acupoint. To increase the pressure, you can use one finger pressing on another. Use your palm or elbow to press more muscular parts of the body, such as the back and buttocks.

There are two ways to apply pressure. You can start pressing gently and gradually press harder until your partner feels quite an intense pressure – a feeling that should only last for a moment. Alternatively, you can apply continuous moderate pressure. Take care not to press too roughly or too hard.

Kneading

This technique exerts a firm, steady pressure in a circular manner. Use either your finger, palm, heel of the palm, side of the thumb, thumb, or elbow to knead an acupoint or area. Knead first in a clockwise circle, and then anticlockwise, gradually increasing the pressure applied and then reducing it again.

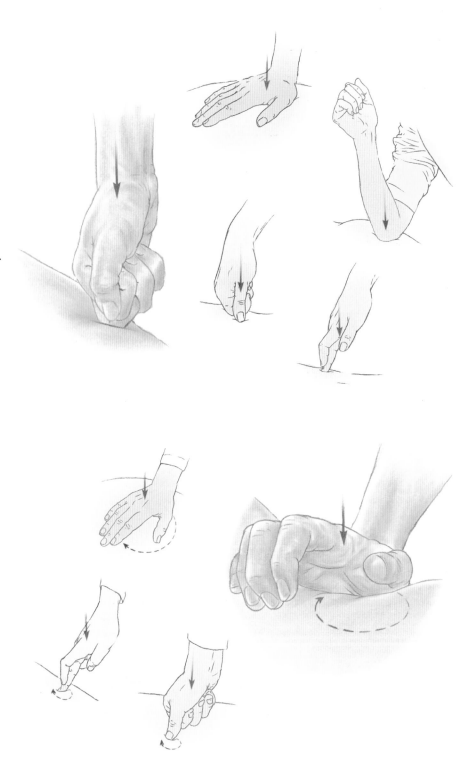

Pinching

Pinch an acupoint or area between the tip of your thumb and the tips of your index and middle fingers. Pinch firmly and hold with continuous, forceful pressure. Your partner will feel sore and feel some pain as you pinch, but this should soon subside. However, take care not to exceed your partner's pain threshold, or to damage the skin.

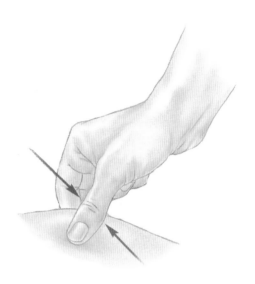

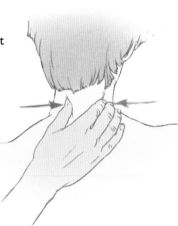

Squeezing

This technique can be used on most parts of the body. Make a "pincer" shape with your thumb, index, and middle fingers, or with your thumb and all four fingers for squeezing larger areas. Repeatedly squeeze and release, keeping your wrist relaxed and the squeezing action slow and rhythmic. Gradually increase the force you apply and then reduce it again.

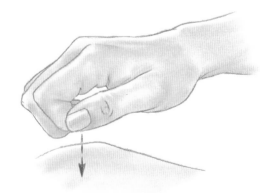

Percussing

Clench your fist loosely and use the flattened finger surface (not the knuckles) to tap gently and rhythmically, keeping your wrist relaxed and flexible. This technique is used mainly on the legs, shoulders, and back.

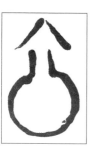

SHIATSU

Shiatsu comes from Japan and involves applying pressure on the acupuncture points in order to balance the body's energy and promote good health. Although its name means simply "finger pressure", shiatsu is also applied with other parts of the hand, as well as with the elbows and knees.

This massage art was given its name in the early 20th century, although its origins are ancient. It is a unique combination of classical Oriental medical theory, dating from over 2000 years ago, and a rich tradition of living folk medicine. The basic principles of Oriental medical theory, or Traditional Chinese Medicine, are described on pages 14–15.

KI

Shiatsu is the generic name for a wide variety of techniques, but all practitioners are linked by a common principle, the belief in a vital force, known as Ki (Qi in Chinese), which arises from the interplay between Yin and Yang (see page 14). Ki flows in connected Meridians (or Channels) throughout the body; each Meridian is linked to an organ or psycho-physical function (see page 15). Ki can be contacted at certain points along the Meridians – these are known as acupoints in Chinese medicine (see page 15), and by their Japanese name, Tsubo, in shiatsu. In health, a balanced condition prevails and the Ki flows smoothly along the Meridians, like fuel through a pipeline, supplying and maintaining all parts of the body. But when the body has been weakened by an immoderate lifestyle, emotional stress, or injury, the Ki no longer flows smoothly, becoming deficient in some areas and excessive in others.

The shiatsu Meridians are based on the Channels in Chinese Medicine, though some extend further. Your shiatsu will be effective if you treat the Channels shown on pages 240–41, since working on part of a Meridian tonifies and/or releases the whole Meridian.

GIVING SHIATSU

In shiatsu you are aiming to treat the cause of your partner's symptoms. To treat only the head for a headache is to ignore one of the fundamental principles of Oriental medicine – that body and mind are an indivisible, organic whole. To diagnose the exact cause of a person's symptoms requires both a thorough grasp of Oriental medical theory and an understanding of that person's emotional and psychological condition. Unless you have those skills, it is more effective to treat the whole body.

With practice you will learn to sense by touch the areas which show an excess of Ki, called Jitsu, and those where Ki is deficient, called Kyo. Usually the Jitsu or painful area is the symptom, and the Kyo area the cause, so you will treat most effectively if you concentrate on Kyo areas in your shiatsu. A little background knowledge, the time to give a full-body treatment, attention and sensitivity toward your partner – this is all you need to begin to feel your way toward a real understanding of shiatsu.

Kyo and Jitsu

In a Meridian which is out of balance, Ki can be either deficient (Kyo) or in excess (Jitsu), and sometimes, when Ki flow is obstructed, it can be both at once – in excess above the obstruction and deficient below it. Kyo areas often look and feel slightly hollow and are usually yielding to the touch. When you press a Kyo Meridian it generally feels good to your partner, as you are supplying Ki to a deficiency. Jitsu areas are easier to find, as they are usually hard or tense. They may be constantly painful, or only when pressed. The pain is generally sharp, whereas the Kyo pain is usually dull and gives relief when you press it – "a good pain".

Shiatsu is far more pleasant and effective when you concentrate on the Kyo areas. This technique, known as "tonification", uses slow and gradual pressure to impart energy to the deficiency. Every excess symptom is caused by a deficiency, so tonifying the Kyo Meridians will help the Jitsu ones to relax.

BASIC STROKES

The illustrations on this page show the basic shiatsu pressure techniques. In shiatsu, you apply pressure by leaning in and letting your body weight do the work for you, rather than by pushing or pressing. To apply stationary pressure, simply lean in your body weight and remain still. The Ki will respond, because its nature is to move. To apply perpendicular pressure, keep a right angle between the direction of your pressure and your partner's body.

Stretches and rotations are also an important part of shiatsu technique, for loosening the joints and smoothing the flow of Ki. These are described in detail in the step-by-step instructions for the whole-body treatment (pages 92–127).

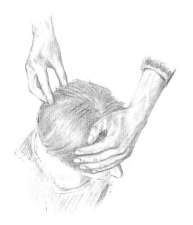

Finger pressure

Finger pressure is often used on delicate areas such as the face. The thumb and finger can be used together when two close points are treated at once.

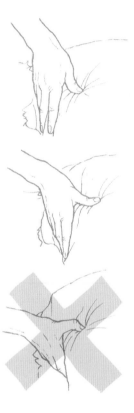

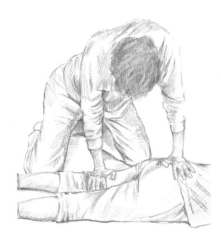

Palm pressure

This technique is used to give gentle but firm pressure over a large area. Place your palm on your partner's body and lean in. Then lean back, slide your palm a little further along, following the shape of your partner's body, and lean in again.

Thumb pressure

Apply strong thumb pressure by leaning your weight through the thumb tip, or for gentler pressure hold the ball of the thumb more flat. Always use the thumb extended, so it continues the line of your arm, and is not bent. Steady the thumb by extending your fingers to support your hand – never use the thumb on its own.

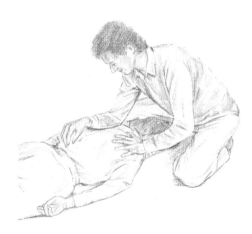

Elbow pressure

Elbows are excellent for working into stiff or painful muscles associated with tension. First use your fingers to feel the shape and condition of the area you are working on, then locate your elbow comfortably. Hold your arm open at the elbow and lean in on the flattened underside of the angle, not the point.

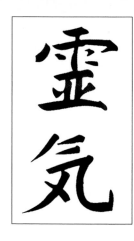

REIKI

Reiki is one of the most ancient healing methods. It originated in Tibet and was rediscovered in the 19th century by a Japanese monk, Dr Mikao Usui. The tradition of Reiki is referred to in 2500-year-old writings in Sanskrit, the ancient Indian language. The Usui System of Natural Healing, named after Dr Usui, has been passed down by Reiki Masters since that time and is today practised worldwide.

Universal Life Energy is all around us and within us. In the Japanese word "rei-ki", "rei" describes the cosmic, universal aspect of this energy and "ki" the fundamental life force flowing and pulsating in all living things. This life force energy is given to us at birth. We bring with us a certain amount of "ki" to life and use it up in the business of ordinary daily living. We then have to replenish this supply, from the food we eat and the air we breathe. When we are unable to make up for our energy consumption for a prolonged period, we may become physically or emotionally ill. If our supply of life force energy is extremely low and depleted, we suffer from physical, emotional, and mental exhaustion and tend to be much more irritable, bad-tempered, and depressed than usual.

In a Reiki treatment, the giver lightly places his or her hands in particular positions on the receiver's body and holds them there, connecting with Universal Life Energy and drawing it through and into the giver and receiver. When you give Reiki, you can focus your intention by visualizing a beam of energy, in the form of a healing light, flowing down from the universe, through you, and out of your hands into your partner. While the Universal Life Energy flows through you, the giver, during the treatment, it also fortifies and harmonizes you at the same time.

Reiki works at a cellular level, speeding renewal and regeneration, so people who give or receive regular Reiki tend to have more energy on a day-to-day basis. It works directly according to the intention of the giver, even when you treat yourself.

Reiki can be learned by all who open themselves to it. It offers a wide-ranging insight into the various areas of the human experience – physical, mental, emotional, and spiritual. Reiki not only promotes your physical wellbeing but also has a positive effect on your emotional and spiritual equilibrium. After a treatment with Reiki, many people feel refreshed, relaxed, clearer, and more content in themselves.

Attunements

The key to Reiki is provided by "energy attunements", which differentiate Reiki from other healing methods. These attunements enable you to allow the Life Force Energy to flow through you more intensely. When you train with a Reiki Master you receive one or more attunements, depending on which Reiki Degree you are training in. Attunement usually takes place during a simple ceremony, where the Reiki Master attunes each person individually into the Reiki healing method. Using an ancient Tibetan technique, the Master transmits energy to the students, using the confidential Reiki symbols and mantras to amplify the flow.

The attunements open your inner healing channel, allowing more Universal Life Energy to flow through you. At each attunement, a kind of cleansing takes place on a physical, emotional, mental, and spiritual level. The attunements release blocks in you and toxins are set free. You can, however, give the Reiki treatments described in this book without having attuned to Reiki. You will still channel the energy to the receiver, but at a lower intensity.

BREATHING EXERCISE

To experience some of the power of Reiki, try this relaxation exercise.

Step 1
Make yourself comfortable lying on your back and close your eyes. Pay attention to your breath and follow its rhythm. Notice how it flows in and out.

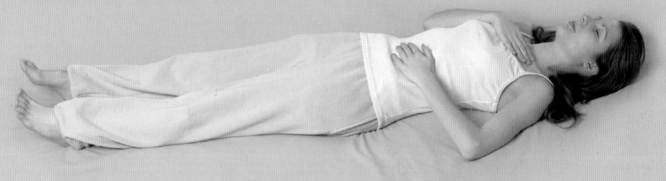

Step 2
Now put your hands on your body wherever you feel drawn to, or where you feel tension. Use your intuition to locate the spot in your body that needs relaxation the most.

Step 3
Now direct your breath consciously and repeatedly to this place. Imagine that your breath is the Universal Life Energy which flows through you. Let it collect and expand under your hands. Notice how a feeling of relaxation and peace gradually spreads from that place throughout your entire body.

Step 4
After about 5 minutes, place your hand on another part of your body. Again, breathe into your hands. You may find that your breath changes in some positions, as you awaken memories and experiences that are stored there. You need not consciously probe feelings or initiate stronger breathing. Just allow yourself to let go and to plunge into this feeling of flowing.

Step 5
Move on to two further places on your body, and charge them with energy. Then slowly open your eyes, stretch, and return to your normal daytime consciousness, feeling calmer, relaxed, and more centred.

AROMATHERAPY MASSAGE

Like herbalism, aromatherapy draws on the healing power of the plant world, but instead of using the whole or part of a plant it employs only its essential oil. This potent, aromatic substance is housed in tiny glands on the outside or deep inside the roots, wood, leaves, flowers, or fruit of a plant. It is a dynamic, concentrated representation of the healing properties of the plant, which some believe contains its life force.

Aromatic herbs have been used since ancient times to cleanse and heal both body and mind. In the East, primitive stills were in use 5000 years ago, although probably more for the production of aromatic waters than for essential oils. In ancient Egypt, aromatic waters and resins featured in ceremonies and rituals, and oils of cedarwood and frankincense were used in the embalming process. Ayurvedic medical texts from early Indian society include aromatic essences in many of their treatments. Subsequent societies, notably the Greeks and Romans, developed the use of these essences in rituals and religious ceremonies and records demonstrate an increasing awareness of their therapeutic properties. By the 11th century AD, the Arab physician Avicenna had introduced the cooling system into the distillation process, making the extraction of essential oils more efficient.

An indication of the antiseptic properties of essential oils came from the apparent immunity of the perfumers to the plagues and cholera that swept through Europe in the Middle Ages, and by the late 17th century the oils were widely used in medicine. Toward the end of the 19th century, scientific experiments into the anti-bacterial properties of plants began to clarify the chemical composition and potential healing powers of essential oil molecules. However, this led to the development of synthetic chemical equivalents, rather than an increased use of plant essences.

Early in the 20th century a French chemist, René-Maurice Gattefossé, working with essential oils, first coined the name "aromathérapie" for this branch of herbalism. Later another Frenchman, Dr Jean Valnet, became interested in the healing properties of essential oils after using them to treat soldiers' wounds in World War II. This led to official recognition for the therapy in France, where many doctors prescribe oils for internal and external use.

Aromatherapy massage developed from the work of French biochemist Margaret Maury, who introduced essential oils into beauty therapy, where they were used in conjunction with massage for their rejuvenating effects on the skin.

AROMATHERAPY AND YOUR HEALTH

In aromatherapy massage, the essential oil is diluted in a carrier oil and massaged into the skin, where it is thought to permeate through to the capillaries and cell tissues. Since essential oils evaporate readily on exposure to air, they are also absorbed into the olfactory system by inhalation during the massage. This triggers the release of neurochemicals in the brain, which may be sedative, relaxing, stimulating, or euphoric in effect. Once within your system, the essential oils work to re-establish harmony and revitalize those systems or organs where there is a malfunction or lack of balance. Each oil has its own particular qualities (see the chart on page 250), but they are noted in particular for their antiseptic properties and their ability to restore balance to body and mind.

Neat essential oils are powerful, concentrated substances. Prior to use on the skin they are normally diluted in a carrier oil or lotion (see page 29) to facilitate application and to ensure that there is no adverse skin reaction.

BASIC STROKES

For aromatherapy massage, the basic strokes are kneading, gliding, and friction. Variations on these are described fully in the step-by-step instructions for the whole-body (pages 154–69) and self-massage sequences (pages 208–11).

Kneading

This stroke is used to break down muscle tension and to stimulate circulation. Both hands work together in a rhythmic sequence, alternately picking up and gently squeezing the tense muscle between fingers and palm. As one hand releases the muscle, the other takes over.

Gliding

Use light, long, smooth strokes at the beginning and end of every session and to spread oil evenly over the body. Glide both hands together over the skin, as far as you can reach, then move to the outside and back up your partner's body in a circular sweep, to return to your starting position.

Friction

These strokes, using the heel of the hand, or the pads of the fingers or thumbs, are used to penetrate deep muscle tissue.

Thumb pressure is often most effective for knotted muscles. Use circular pressure on a point, or move the thumb in wider circles.

Caution: *never use this stroke on sciatic pain, since it can irritate the nerve.*

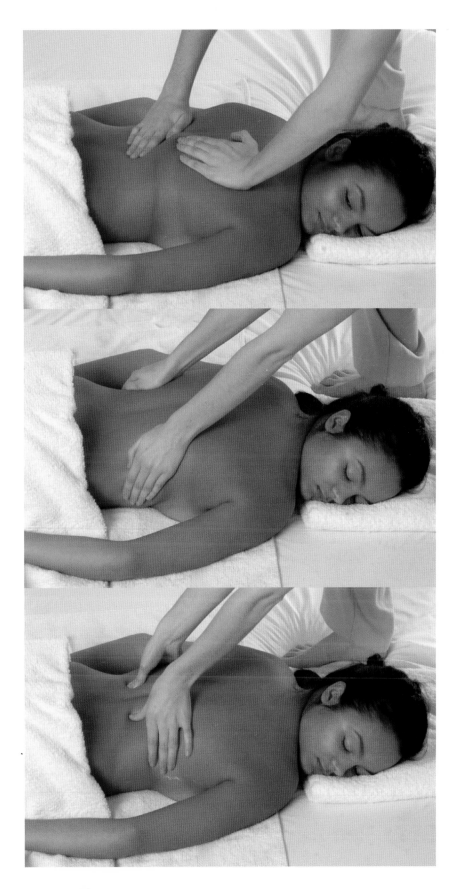

REFLEXOLOGY

Reflexology is a completely safe and non-invasive therapy that works by applying pressure to specific reflex points on the feet and hands. Each reflex point corresponds to a part of the body (see the charts on pages 246–9). Everything on the right side of your body corresponds to reflex points on your right hand or foot, while everything on the left side corresponds to the left hand or foot. Working these reflex points stimulates the nerve endings and blood circulation, as well as alleviating stress and tension held in the body.

Reflexology is centuries old. Wall paintings dating from 2330 BC on the Tomb of the Physicians in Ankomohor, Egypt, are the earliest records of it in use. One scene shows people receiving treatment on their hands and feet. Chinese acupuncturists also used reflexology in the 4th century AD to complement their work. They applied direct pressure to the feet when the needles were in place, to help release energy and induce healing. Eunice Ingham, an American physiotherapist, introduced the West to modern reflexology in the 1930s. She learned about and refined reflexology from ancient foot maps.

Although scientific research has been unable to prove how reflexology, acupuncture, or similar therapies work, cellular memory – the way the brain stores and retrieves information – offers a helpful and credible explanation. Because the brain records all our experiences, it also remembers things that have obviously changed or we think we have forgotten. Physical illness can leave its memory of inflammation, tension, and congestion in the brain cells. In reflexology the congested part of the body manifests itself as sensitive foot and hand reflex points. When these are stimulated, the nervous system sends a new, corrected message to the brain. With frequent treatment the cell memory changes and the function of the body is restored. The reflex points that were previously very sensitive also become non-reactive.

Reflexology can be used in combination with most other practical therapies, such as aromatherapy, massage, Reiki, shiatsu, Chinese massage, acupuncture, or yoga. It is quite safe to have reflexology when you are receiving homeopathy or herbalism, although you should always consult your practitioner first.

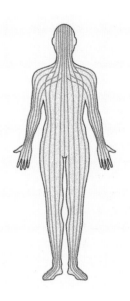

Mapping the zones

The body is divided into ten energy zones, five on each side of the spine. The zones start at the toes, zone 1 starting at the big toe, and run up to the head. The hands also form part of the zone map, with zone 1 starting at the thumb. Any condition interrupting the flow of energy through a given zone will disturb the healthy functioning of the body parts lying along it. For the first zonal pair, this would include the spine, neck, and brain. In the same way, when you apply pressure to the hands and feet the whole zone is stimulated and its healing effect is felt throughout the whole body.

BASIC STROKES

The two basic techniques used in reflexology treatments are creeping and rotating. Other techniques are described fully in the step-by-step instructions for the reflexology foot treatment (pages 170–81) and the self-massage treatment for the hands (pages 212–17).

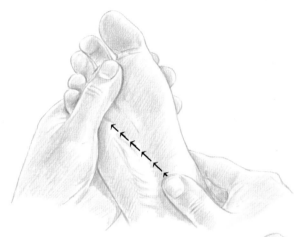

Hands or feet?

Reflexology is most effective when given to the feet, as they are more sensitive. Try dipping first your hands and then your feet into a hot bath – you will find that a temperature that is bearable for your hands will be too hot for your feet. Also, the reflexes are harder to isolate on the hands than on the feet, as the surface area of the hands is much smaller. However, a hand treatment is ideal for self-help when you do not have a willing partner to give you the full foot treatment.

Creeping

The forward-creeping motion of this technique is similar to how a caterpillar moves. Keep your thumb (or finger) flexed and work with the flat pad, pressing down slightly on the outer edge so that the nail does not dig in. Release the pressure, slide your thumb forward a little and repeat. It is a tiny action that lets you work slowly and methodically.

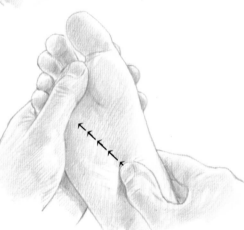

Rotating

When the kidney, adrenal, eye, and ear reflex points on the toes need extra stimulation, use the rotation technique. Place the flat of your thumb on the appropriate reflex point and rotate it inward, toward the spine, using a small but firm movement. For maximum benefit, maintain the pressure for several seconds.

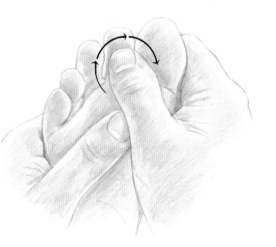

HEAD MASSAGE

Good health depends on balanced energy. This energy, called Qi or Ki in Oriental medicine, or Prana in Indian tradition, is the life force itself. It permeates our bodies and every living thing in the universe. When our energy is unbalanced we may feel irritable, out of sorts, or even seriously unwell.

Stress, poor diet, strong emotions, or toxin build-up are all symptoms of modern living that can unbalance life energy and create areas of negativity. The power of energy healing lies in rebalancing the life force so that the flow of energy within us is constant, effortless, and unblocked. Head massage provides a simple and effective way to rebalance your energies and clear any areas of negativity, easing and even preventing illness.

Many of the head massage techniques in this book are based on traditional Indian head massage. Some are drawn from other ancient and traditional methods of healing, such as shiatsu, Reiki, Chinese massage, and Qi Gong. Although each uses different terminology to explain the theory, all of these methods are based on a common concept: that life energy flows within us, and by working on the channels it flows through, or specific points or areas, this energy can be brought into balance.

Touch alone is very powerful, but another vital ingredient in head massage is the intention of the giver to transmit healing, caring, love, and wellbeing to the receiver.

BASIC STROKES

Practise the basic head massage techniques described here before giving the head massage treatment (pages 182–95) or using the self-massage sequence (pages 218–23). Any additional techniques used are described fully in the step-by-step instructions for these sequences.

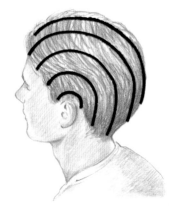

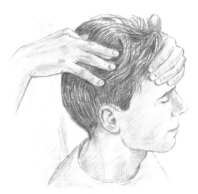

Working in lines

For many head massage techniques, such as rotations and finger pressure, you will need to work in lines over the head.

Begin with your left hand, working back along a line from the hairline in the centre of the forehead, to the nape of the neck, moving your finger position back two finger widths each time. Now place your finger on the hairline two finger widths to the left of your first line and work back in a line parallel to the first. Continue to work lines in this way until you have covered the left half, finishing with a line running just above the ear. Stroke the hair gently, then use your right hand to work back in lines on the right side of the head.

Finger kneading

Use your middle finger to press on your index finger and knead by pressing firmly and then releasing, rhythmically and evenly, for 3–5 seconds on each point. Work back over the head in lines, as for rotations.

Pressure

For this technique you can use your fingers, thumbs, hands, or elbows, and lean in with your body weight to vary the amount of pressure used. When working on a very tense area, a continuous whole-body rocking action of pressure and release is very effective. Alternatively, apply stationary pressure for 3–5 seconds before moving to the next point.

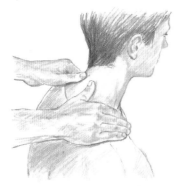

Thumb pressure

Use your thumbs to apply strong pressure to the upper back, shoulders, and neck. Start with your thumbs either side of the spine, level with the bottom of the shoulder blades. Lean forward, with your weight on your thumbs, hold for 3–5 seconds and then release. Move your thumbs two finger widths outward, then lean in again. Repeat, moving two finger widths out along this horizontal line each time, until you come to the edges of the back.

Starting either side of the spine again, two finger widths up from your first line, work a parallel line. Repeat until you reach the neck.

Caution: *do not massage the back of the neck on anyone who has cancer.*

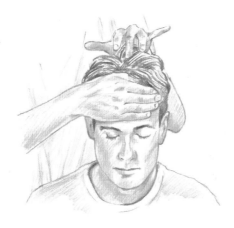

Rotations

This technique should be used in a slow, meditative way. You can use one or more fingers, your thumbs, the heel of your hand, or your whole hand. To support your partner's head while you work, cup your non-working hand on the forehead, taking care not to push down on the eyebrows. For one finger rotations, place the pad of your index or middle finger in the centre of the forehead at the hairline. Using firm pressure, rotate your finger for 3–5 seconds. Then move your finger two finger widths back along the midline and repeat the rotation. Continue until you reach the nape of the neck. Work over the whole head in lines.

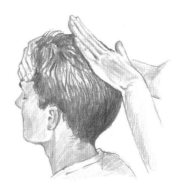

Heel of hand kneading

Support the forehead carefully with one hand. Place the heel of the other at the nape of the neck, applying pressure while rolling from the heel up over the palm to the fingertips. Work up to the front of the head along the midline, then work up the sides in the same way, starting at the nape each time.

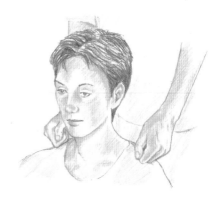

Knuckling

Curl your hands into fists and rest them on the shoulders. Rock your fists back and forth, from the little finger to the index finger and back again, with firm and steady pressure. Move slowly along the shoulders. This stimulating technique can also be used on the head and neck.

Caution: *do not massage the midpoint of the shoulders on anyone who is pregnant.*

GIVING MASSAGE

Care and sensitivity, a little time and energy, and a good pair of hands – that is all you need to begin practising massage. However, it is worth taking some time to prepare both yourself and the room for the session, whichever of the massage treatments you are giving. How you begin and end the treatment is also important.

CREATING A RELAXING ENVIRONMENT

For a massage session the room should be warm and snug, with pillows, cushions, blankets, towels, and any oil you may need to hand. You will break the flow of the treatment if you have to stop to go and fetch another heater or more oil, and your partner will be unable to relax during the massage if he is chilly or uncomfortable. Choose a time when you are unlikely to be interrupted and turn off the telephone, so that your concentration remains unbroken. Some people like to play soothing background music, others may find music of any kind intrusive. The lighting in the room should be soft and subdued – the glow of candlelight is ideal. As a final touch, you may wish to use flowers or incense to add fragrance to the atmosphere.

THE WORKING SURFACE

Holistic, aromatherapy, and intuitive massage can be given on a massage table or on the floor, while shiatsu, Chinese massage and Reiki are traditionally given on the floor. If your floor is well carpeted, you need only spread out a folded blanket or duvet for the receiver. But if the floor is hard you will need extra padding, such as a futon or thin piece of foam. Make sure that the padding extends beyond your partner's body, to save your knees as you move around. If you are using oil in your massage, it is a good idea to protect your working area with a sheet or towel.

For head massage and some steps in Chinese massage your partner will need to sit in an upright chair. For a reflexology treatment, the receiver sits with his foot in your lap. You will need a low chair or cushions to sit on, while a comfortable chair will allow your partner to lean back and relax.

PREPARING YOURSELF

Wash your hands and ensure that your fingernails are clean and short; always wash your hands at the end of the session. Wear loose, comfortable clothes that allow you to move freely and remove any jewellery and your watch. Each time you change positions during the session, make sure that you feel relaxed, not strained, before carrying on with the treatment. Never make do with a slightly awkward position, thinking that the discomfort will disappear. It won't, and you will transmit your tension to your partner. Your comfort is closely linked to your posture and breathing; whether you are sitting, kneeling, or standing, your body should feel balanced and relaxed. If you can breathe fully and let your body "dance" as you move, you will avoid getting tense and will end a treatment with as much energy as when you started.

Before giving a treatment, talk to the receiver and find out if there are any special problems. Encourage him to tell you during the session if he is ever uncomfortable or if your pressure is too light or too strong. Never attempt to give a treatment if you are upset, angry, or unwell – your energy will be depleted and your mood will affect your partner.

GIVING AND RECEIVING

Massage is a two-way flow of touch and response, a mutual exchange of energy. The terms "giver" and "receiver" are deceptive, since any form of touch therapy is a matter for sharing. For the healing power of touch to come through, both need to understand their roles in the exchange. Both need to give and to be receptive – the receiver by giving his trust, by surrendering to the giver; the giver by being open and sensitive to the receiver's needs.

PREPARING AND USING OILS

When massaging bare skin, oil allows you to slide your hands smoothly and evenly over the contours without any risk of friction or jerkiness. It also nourishes the skin. Only a thin film is sufficient to lubricate the skin; too much oil prevents you making proper contact. Since most oils are quickly absorbed by the skin, oil

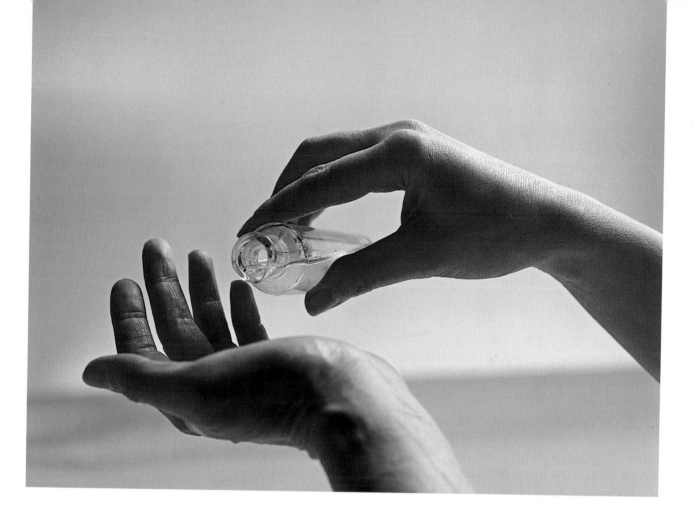

each separate part of the body as you begin to work on it. Begin the massage treatment by centring yourself (see page 30), then let your hands rest briefly on your partner's head or body for the first gentle contact. Pour about half a teaspoon of oil into one palm, then rub your palms together to spread the oil before applying it to your partner's body using long, sweeping strokes.

There is no need to buy ready-made massage oils – use a light vegetable oil, such as grapeseed, sunflower, safflower, or almond. You can also use mineral oils, such as baby oil, but these are less easily absorbed. To scent your massage oil, or for aromatherapy massage, add essential oils to the base oil. To choose a suitable essential oil, consult the chart on page 250. Neat essential oils are very powerful, concentrated substances that need to be diluted in a carrier oil before application to the skin. Add 20 drops of essential oil to 60 ml (2 fl oz or 10 tsp) of carrier oil in a screw-top bottle, then replace the lid and

shake well. Before giving a massage treatment, warm the oil by standing the bottle in a bowl of hot water.

TOWELS

When receiving a massage, there is nothing more comforting and relaxing than having a soft, warmed towel placed gently over your body. In a professional massage session, towels are always used to cover the parts of the body not being worked on, for the sake of privacy and warmth. At home, elaborate towel technique is probably unnecessary, although the receiver will often relax more deeply if only half the body is exposed at a time.

You will need two bath towels, which you should warm on a radiator before use. You should also have a smaller hand towel available for women who prefer their breasts to be covered while you massage the front of the torso. At the beginning of the massage, with the receiver lying on his front, place one towel lengthwise covering the buttocks and legs, and another horizontally across the shoulders and upper back. When you begin the massage on the shoulders and upper back, simply remove the upper towel.

The basic principle is to uncover only the part of the body you are going to massage next, and cover it again when you have finished. The holistic and aromatherapy whole-body sequences include notes on how to arrange the towels when necessary. The way you move and arrange the towels requires the same sensitivity and awareness that you bring to the massage, so avoid throwing towels carelessly over the receiver's body, or pulling them off suddenly.

BEGINNING AND ENDING THE SESSION

Most massage therapies recommend that you begin the treatment by centring yourself, and connecting with your partner's energies, and end the treatment similarly by disconnecting.

Centring meditation

Sit cross-legged or kneel on the floor, or sit on a straight-backed chair with both feet flat on the floor. Now close your eyes and direct your attention inward. Feel the strong foundation of your buttocks, legs, and feet as they make contact with the chair or floor. From this firm base, allow your spine to float gently upward, without strain. Let go of any tension in your shoulders, neck, and face. Now begin to focus on your breath, allowing it to find its own rhythm. Imagine that as you inhale, your breath fills your lower abdomen or Hara. After a few breaths, begin also to visualize that, as you exhale, your breath flows up your torso from the Hara, through your shoulders, down your arms, and out of your hands.

Remaining centred

For all touch therapies, it is essential to keep your attention in the "here and now", for the healing energy transmitted through your hands will be weakened or deflected by an absent mind. When you are centred, you are guided by your intuition and will more readily sense where the sources of tension or energy imbalance lie in your partner. If your thoughts

Cleansing visualization

This simple visualization will cleanse the energy of the space you are working in, creating a healing space filled with protective energy.

Sit for a few moments in the middle of the space. Close your eyes and visualize a gold ring spinning just above your head. Watch it growing larger and descending so that it comes down around your body, leaving behind a golden trace as it descends, enveloping you in a bubble. Watch the energy within this bubble turn to a soft pink, and move this energy outward from you until it fills the whole room.

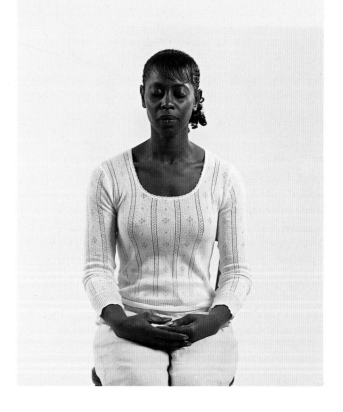

start to drift, simply bring them back and quieten your mind by concentrating on your breathing. Working with your eyes closed for brief periods may help you stay in touch with what you are doing and keep your attention in your hands.

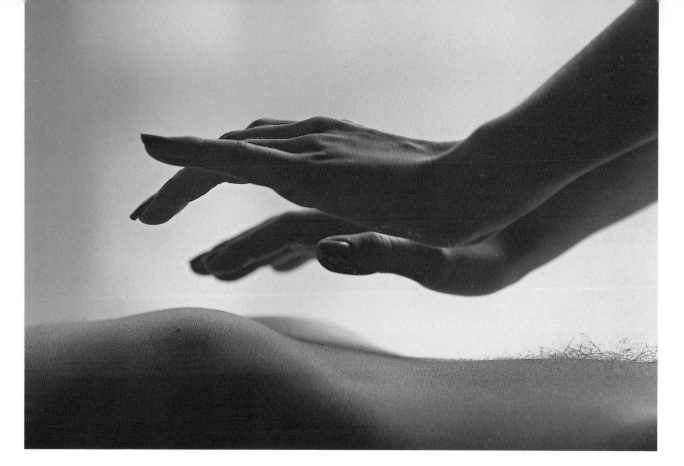

Making the energy connection

Before you start the massage, stand or kneel quietly with your palms facing downward, thumbs together, flat on your partner's body. Allow your breathing to synchronize as you make contact with his energies. Close your eyes and visualize a pink healing light coming from the universe down into your head, flowing down your body into your Hara and then back up your body, along your arms, and through your hands into your partner. Watch this energy moving in a great circle from the heavens, through you both, down into the earth, and then back up to the stars. Try to maintain contact with this energy throughout the massage.

Breaking the energy connection

At the end of the massage, hold your partner's head firmly but gently, with your hands on either side. Close your eyes and again visualize the pink healing light moving in a circle through you and your partner, down into the earth, then back up to the stars. Now see this flow of light being cut above your head. Remove your hands from your partner, holding them 2–3 cm (1 in) above her head. See the light flowing down through your body, through your partner, out through the bottom of your feet, and into the earth. Move back away from your partner, take some deep breaths and shake your hands vigorously. This breaks the energy connection between you.

Clearing visualization

At the end of the massage, after you have broken contact with your partner, use this visualization to clear your energy and the energy of the space.

Slowly bring the bubble in around you until it is about 5 cm (2 in) from your body. See the gold ring spinning beneath you. Move the ring up through your body until it is above your head. Feel the energy rising up through your body with the gold ring. Then watch the ring grow smaller and slowly rise up out of sight.

CHAPTER 2

HOLISTIC MASSAGE

This whole-body sequence starts on the back, working down from the head to the feet. Because you reach nerves on the back that spread to every part of the body, most people feel a deep sense of release after a thorough back massage. By the time you come to work on the more "vulnerable" parts of the body, your partner will generally be feeling more trusting and relaxed. The receiver then turns over and the massage continues on the front of the body, again working down from head to foot.

Whichever part of the body you are working on, the strokes follow roughly the same order. First you oil the part of the body thoroughly, then work from lighter, broader strokes to the deeper, more specific ones, ending once more with the lighter ones. After working on each part of the body in turn, you use long, flowing connecting strokes to give your partner a sense of wholeness.

Before starting the massage, familiarize yourself with the basic strokes illustrated on pages 12–13. Then prepare the room and yourself for the massage, and warm your massage oil and towels, following the guidelines on pages 28–30. If you are using towels, notes throughout the sequence tell you which parts to cover and uncover. Begin the massage by centring yourself (see page 30). You may also wish to use the cleansing visualization on page 30, or make the energy connection between you (see page 31).

The basic whole-body massage sequence presented here is divided into sections for parts of the body in order to help you learn, but it is not meant to be adhered to rigidly. While giving the massage, ask the receiver for feedback on what feels good, but avoid too much verbal communication as talking will take your concentration away from your hands. The slower and more rhythmical your strokes are, the more relaxed and safe your partner will feel.

Caution: *See page 5 for a full list of cautions and contraindications for massage.*

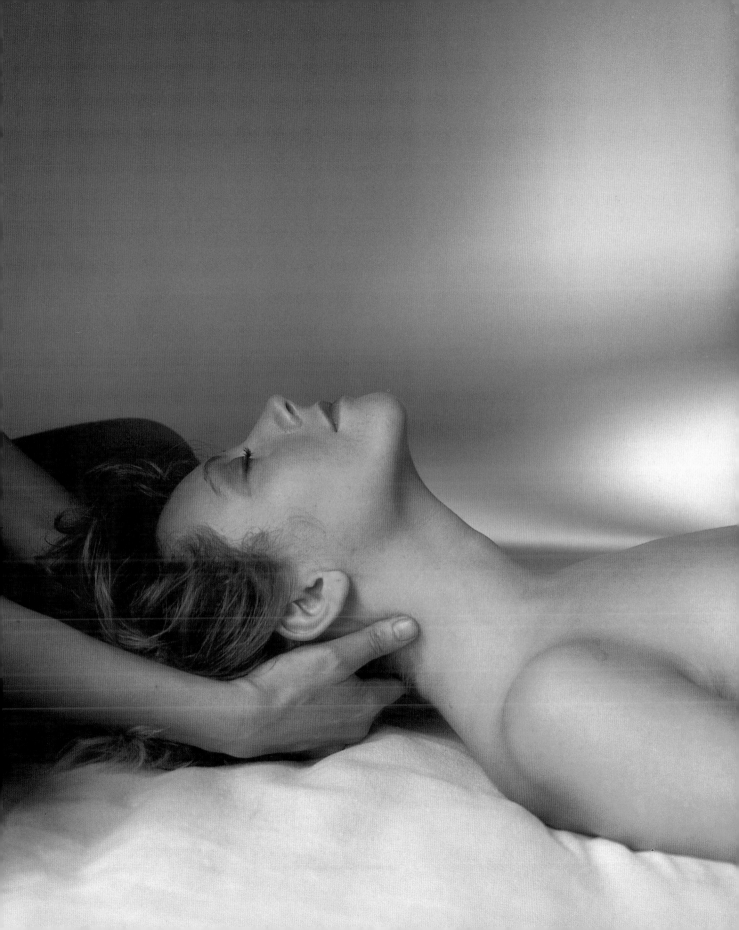

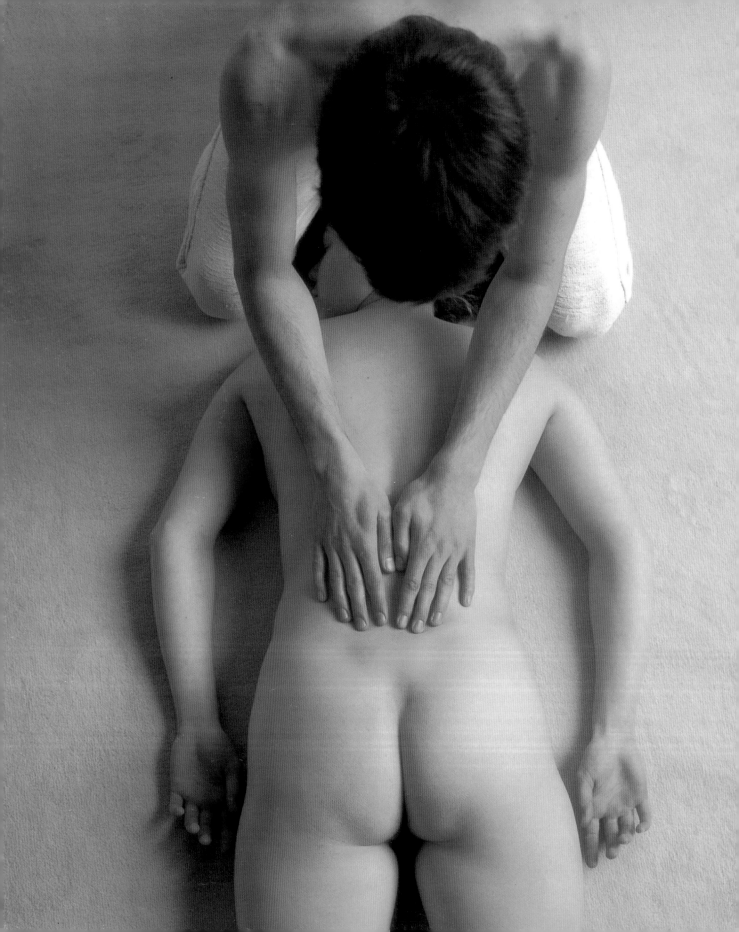

SHOULDERS, NECK, AND BACK

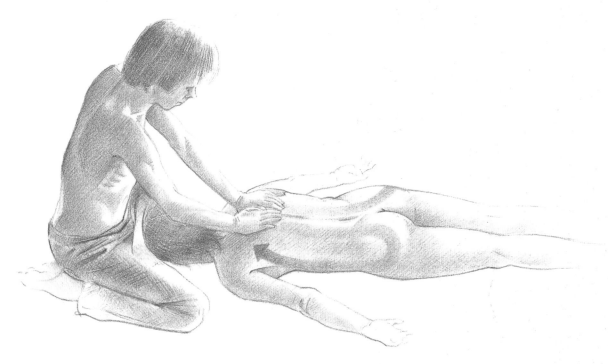

If using towels, cover the buttocks and legs.

Step 1

To massage the back, lie your partner down on her stomach, arms by her sides. Pad under the ankles and, if your partner's neck is a bit stiff, under the upper chest as well. If there is lower back pain, place a pillow under the hips.

Now position yourself at your partner's head and spend a few minutes centring yourself before beginning the long oiling stroke. With this stroke you not only spread the oil and warm the back, but you also acquaint yourself with the receiver's body. As you move slowly over the body, shut your eyes and feel the range of sensations beneath your hands – the softness of the skin, the shape of the bones and muscles, the tightness and tension. Let your stroking be an exploration.

Step 2

Bring your hands down gently on to the upper back; then, rocking forward from the hips, begin to travel down the centre, along each side of the spinal column. At the base of the spine, let your hands divide and curve around to the sides of the buttocks; then rock back, pulling slowly up the sides, across the shoulders. Repeat until the back is thoroughly oiled.

SHOULDERS, NECK, AND BACK

Step 3

Begin with the shoulder that your
partner's head is facing away from.
Using alternate hands, rhythmically
squeeze and gather pockets of flesh.
Knead around the blade and along
this side of the ribcage, as well as
on the shoulder itself, letting your
hands follow the contours.

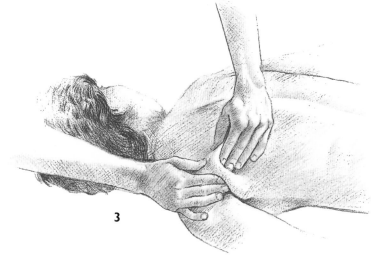

Step 4

Start to work more deeply with
thumb-rolling strokes in the fleshy
triangle at the top of the shoulder
and the base of your partner's neck.
Use small, firm strokes, working
increasingly deeply to release any
tension. Check that your pressure is
acceptable to your partner. Dwell
on any little knots of tension you
may find, interspersing this more
concentrated work with soothing,
broader strokes.

Step 5

Beginning at the base of the neck,
push your thumbs alternately along
the groove beside the spine with
short, firm strokes. Travel down to
the middle of the back, then glide
your hands back to the base of the
neck and repeat.

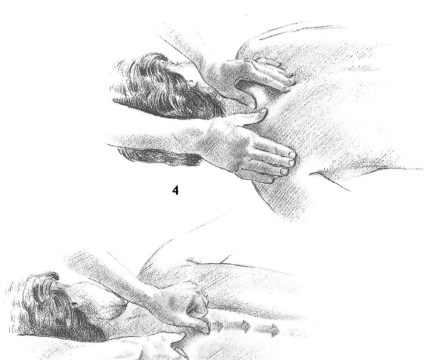

Step 6

Shift your position to work on the same shoulder from the side, facing your partner's head. Lift the forearm carefully on to the lower back, as shown. Cup one hand under the shoulder joint.

Use the fingers of your nearside hand to work around the shoulder blade. Starting at the top, travel slowly down the inner edge of the blade, pushing in firmly under its rim as far as you can. Repeat several times.

Step 7

Now use your fingertips to describe small deep circles on the flat of the blade. Work systematically over the whole area several times.

Step 8

The spine of the shoulder blade runs horizontally across its upper half (A). Once you have located it, work along it a few times from the neck outward, squeezing firmly between fingers and thumb.

Step 9

Grasp the muscles at the base of the neck between the fingers and thumb, and squeeze along them. Then firmly knead the neck itself, thoroughly working the whole area.

Ask your partner to turn his head toward the other shoulder, and repeat steps 1 to 9 on the other side.

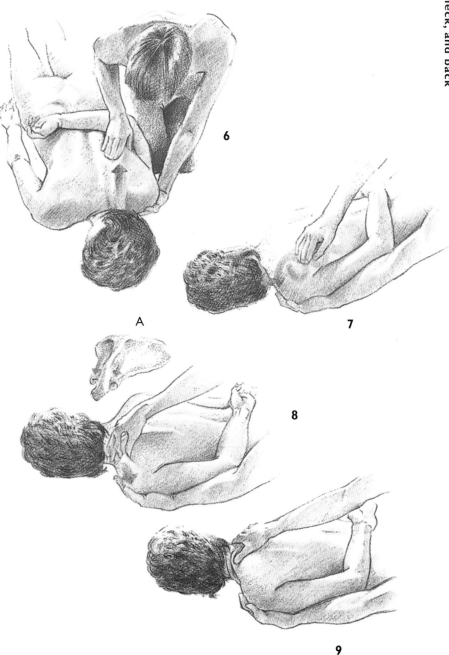

SHOULDERS, NECK AND BACK

If using towels, cover the upper back.

Step 10
Position yourself at your partner's side, level with the thighs. Use alternate hands to circle around the sacrum and lumbar spine (see page 252), using a flat, kneading stroke. Move quite broadly over the whole area, rocking your pelvis from side to side as you circle.

Step 11
Move your hands down to the buttock furthest away from you and begin to knead deeply, gathering parcels of flesh in one hand after the other. Work around the entire buttock, as you squeeze and wring.

Step 12
Still working on the buttock furthest away from you, pick up small pockets of flesh between thumb and fingers, using alternate hands. Try to maintain a fairly rapid but regular rhythm, and keep your hands relaxed and your wrists loose. The flesh should slip easily away through your fingers with each plucking movement.

Step 13
Starting on the buttock furthest away from you, use alternate hands to pull steadily up the far side of the body. Make sure you always have one hand in contact with the body. When you reach the shoulder, use a gliding stroke down that side of the body from shoulder to foot.

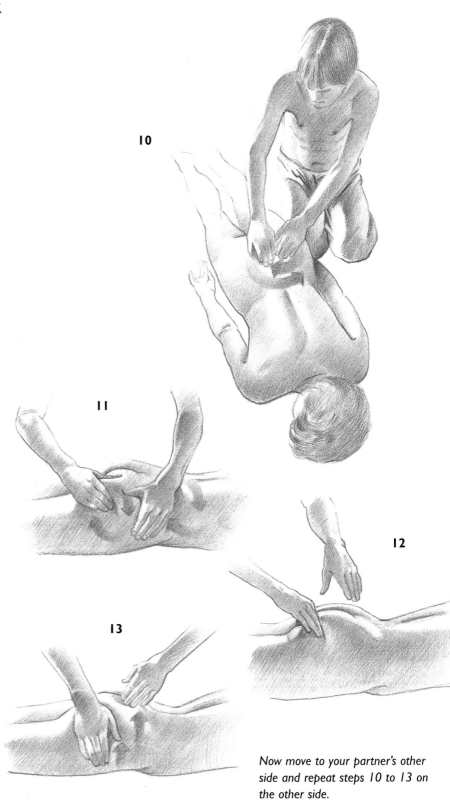

10

11

12

13

Now move to your partner's other side and repeat steps 10 to 13 on the other side.

If using towels, cover the legs.

Step 14
Still at your partner's side, level with the thighs, rest one hand on top of the other and glide both firmly up from the base of the spine to the neck. Using your index and middle fingers (A) press down on either side of the spine, with one hand overlapping the path of the other, so that you ripple gradually down along the whole spine and off at the coccyx.

Step 15
Make small, deep circles with your thumbs up either side of the spine. Avoid pressing directly on the vertebrae and let your hands melt away any knots you find as you work up the back. Press your thumbs briefly into the hollows at the base of the skull, before sweeping lightly back down.

Step 16
Turn to face your partner's side and place your inner forearms in the centre of your partner's back. Slowly pull them apart, bringing one up to the neck, the other to the base of the spine. Repeat, working diagonally across the back, so that one arm goes over one shoulder, the other off the opposite buttock. Repeat, crossing diagonally in the opposite direction.

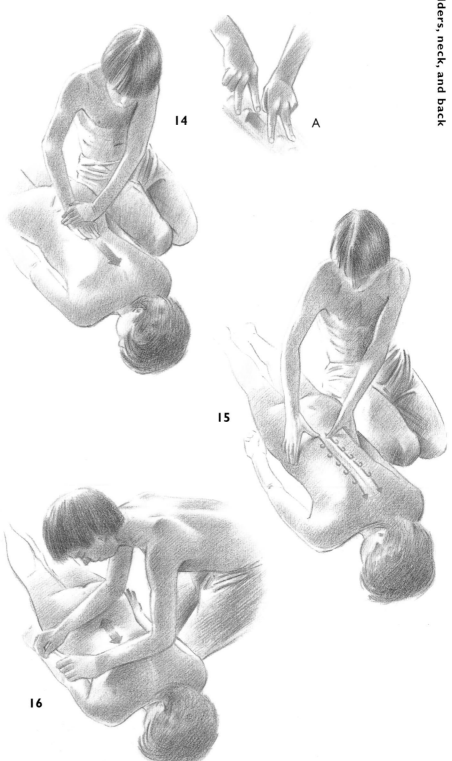

14

A

15

16

BACK OF LEGS

If using towels, cover the back and shoulders.

Caution: *If your partner has varicose veins, avoid all but gentle strokes up the leg, as deep massage may aggravate the condition. Work on either side of the veins and do not stroke down the legs at all.*

Step I
Position yourself between your partner's feet and start by oiling both legs at once, one hand on each leg. If you are working from a kneeling position, rock forward from your hips as you glide up the legs. Oil your hands and let them rest for a moment on the backs of the ankles. Now glide your hands up the centre of your partner's legs – over the buttocks and round the hips, sliding down along the sides of the legs, over the sides of the feet and off the toes. Repeat once or twice.

Now choose which leg you are going to work on first, and position yourself at the foot. The following strokes work with the circulation, assisting the flow of blood back to the heart.

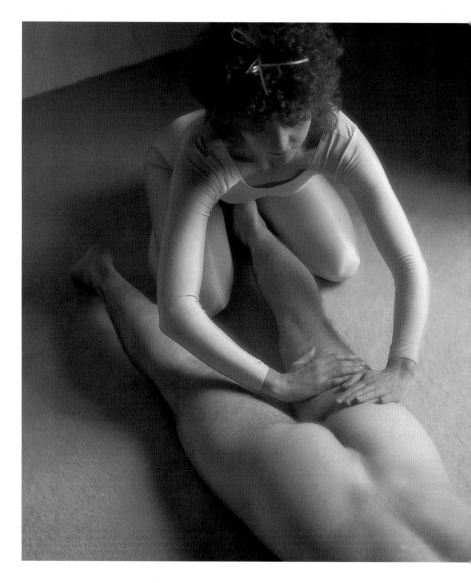

I

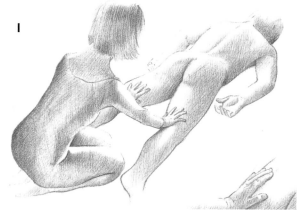

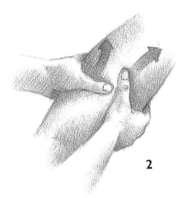

2

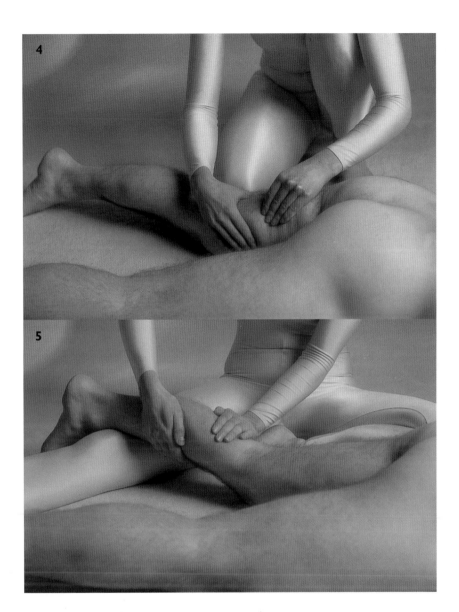

4

5

Step 2

Starting at the ankle, use alternate thumbs to press gradually up the calf and thigh with short, firm strokes. Keep your hands in contact with the leg at all times, to "anchor" your thumbs.

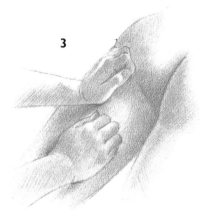

3

Step 3

Starting at the ankle again, work slowly up the leg, pressing with the heels of your hands alternately in broad, deep strokes. Let your movements be continuous and rhythmic and relax your hands. When you come to the back of the knee your strokes should be broader and lighter – if you press too hard, the kneecap will be pushed uncomfortably against the work surface

Step 4

Move to your partner's side and work down the leg from the thigh. Using a rhythmical alternate hand movement, gather and squeeze bunches of flesh over the whole of the thigh and calf. Maintain close contact with the leg – you don't need to lift your hands into the air between handfuls.

Step 5

Starting at the lower calf, wring your hands gradually up and down the back of the leg. Keep your pressure even.

BACK OF LEGS

If using towels, cover the shoulders, back, and buttocks.

Step 6
Place one hand under your partner's ankle and the other on the back of the knee. Slowly lift the lower leg to an upright position.

Step 7
Holding the raised foot firmly with one hand, use the other to work around the ankle bone with fingers or thumb. Loosen around the joint with small circling strokes, first on one side of the leg, then the other.

Step 8
Holding the leg just above the ankle with one hand, grasp the foot with the other and slowly move it around in a wide circle, first in one direction for a few turns, then in the opposite direction. Circle the foot to the limits of its flexibility.

Step 9
Grasp the ankle with one hand and push down on the toes and ball of the foot with the other, flexing the foot as far as its resistance point (A). Then pull the front of the foot back with one hand and push down on the heel with the other, stretching the top of the foot and the front of the leg (B).

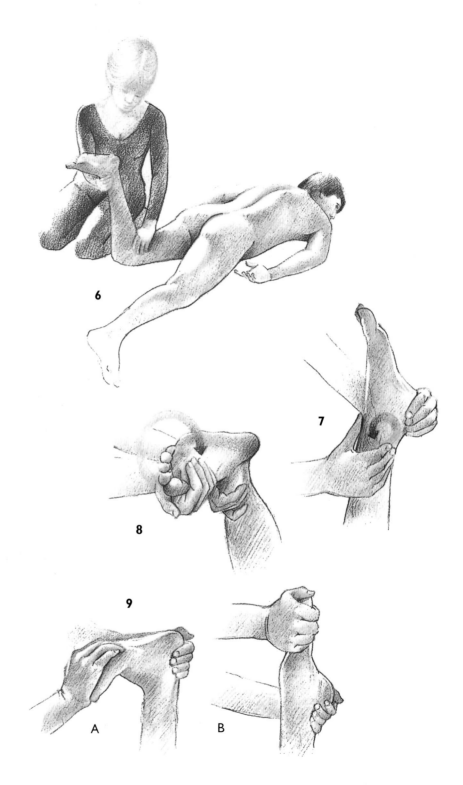

Step 10

With one hand hold the sole of the foot, toes pointing upward. Use the thumb or fingers of your other hand to press slowly along each channel between the tendons on the top of the foot, from ankle to toes.

Step 11

Supporting the foot with one hand, work across the whole of the sole with the thumb of the other hand, making small, firm circling strokes. Start just under the toes and end at the heel.

Step 12

Working systematically along the toes, first stretch them apart sideways, then stretch each toe backward and forward. Be sure to check how far you can stretch the toes with your partner – it is often further than you imagine.

Step 13

One at a time, hold each toe at the base between your thumb and fingers and tug steadily, twisting it a little from side to side as your fingers slide to the tip and off. As you come off each toe, shake your hand, ridding yourself of any negative energy. Lower the leg carefully.

Position yourself at the other foot and repeat steps 2 to 13 on the other leg.

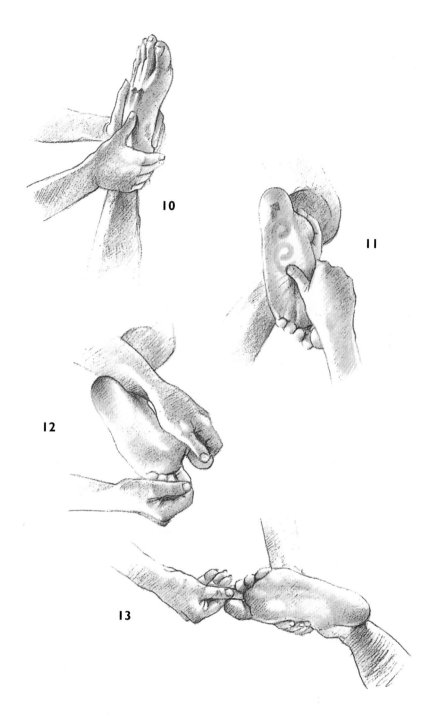

Treating the feet ends the massage on the back of the body. Let your partner rest for a few moments, then ask him to turn over for the massage on the front of the body.

Move the ankle pillow to beneath the knees, and check if he needs a small folded towel under his head.

If using towels, hold them up while the receiver turns over.

NECK, HEAD, BACK, AND SHOULDERS

If using towels, cover the abdomen and legs.

Step 1

Position yourself at your partner's head and begin to apply oil in one continuous long stroke to the whole upper chest, shoulder, and neck area. Place your hands on the upper chest just below the collarbone, fingers pointing toward one another. Slowly draw them apart, heels leading out toward the shoulders (A). As you reach the shoulders, curve your hands round the joints, then slide them along the tops of the shoulders, until you come to the back of the neck (B).

Continue the stroke up the back of the neck to the base of the skull, then up the back of the head and off the crown (C). Repeat the whole stroke a few times.

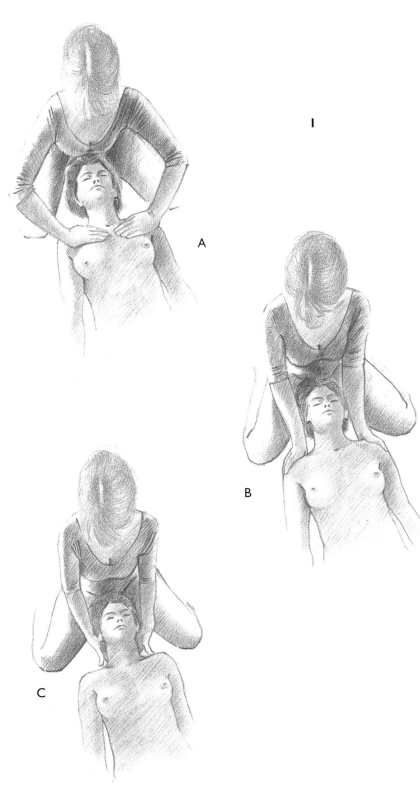

A

B

C

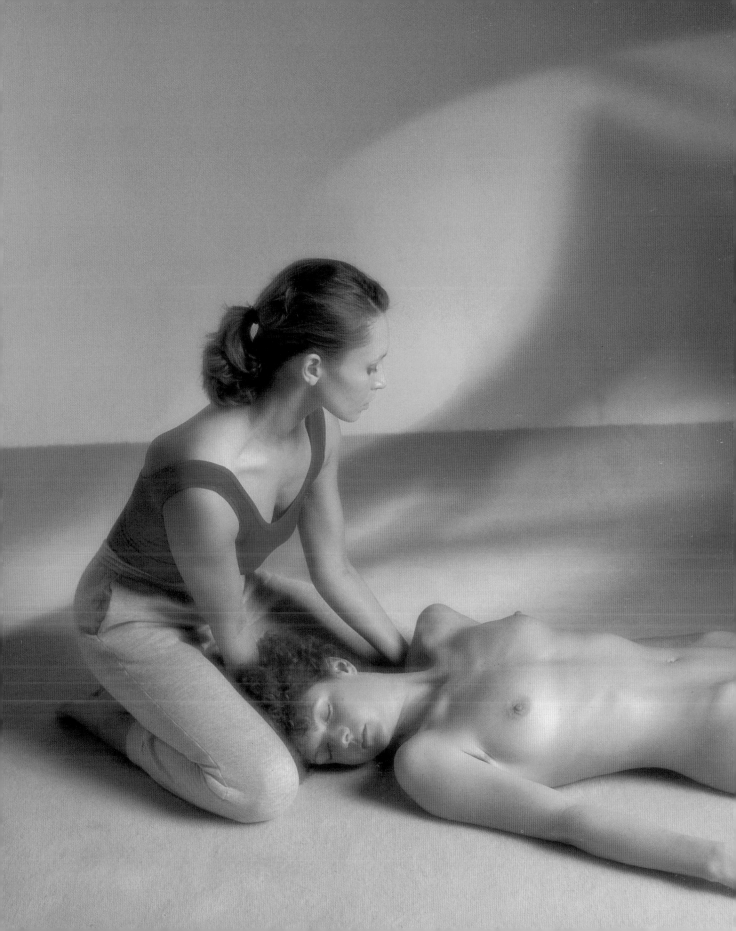

NECK, HEAD, BACK, AND SHOULDERS

Step 2
Cup both hands firmly under the head, fingers at the base of the skull. Lift the head a little way and rock backward, so that you stretch the back of the neck. Lower the head again gently.

Step 3
With your hands still cupped under the head, lift the head up and bring the chin toward the chest (A). Slowly lower the head, then move one hand down to the nape and lift the neck, letting the head tilt right back (B). Now straighten the neck again.

Step 4
Holding the back of the head securely in one hand, "carry" it slowly toward one shoulder while pressing down on the opposite shoulder with the other hand. Bring the head back to the centre, swap hands and repeat on the other side.

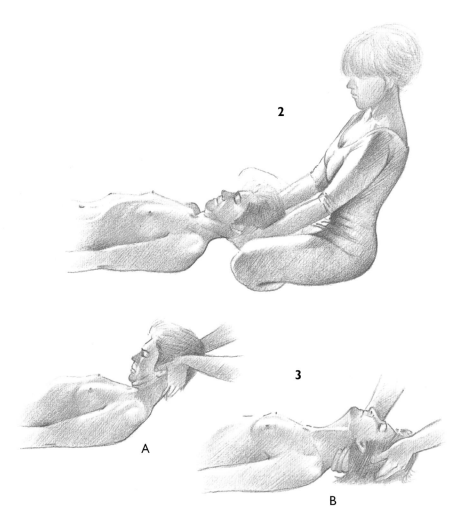

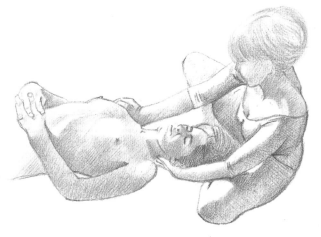

Now you have loosened the whole neck a little, you start to focus on one side at a time. Laying the head on its side on one hand, you use the other hand to work the whole upper back and neck area on the opposite side, following steps 5 and 6, shown on the next page. It is important that you execute this sequence of strokes slowly and with awareness.

Step 5

Hold the head on either side, thumbs just above the ears, fingers behind them. Lift the head slightly and gently turn it to rest on one cupped hand. Check that you are not pulling any hair and that your partner is comfortable.

Step 6

The diagrams illustrate the path of your hands, as much of this sequence takes place out of sight under the back. Begin working on the shoulder your partner is facing away from.

5

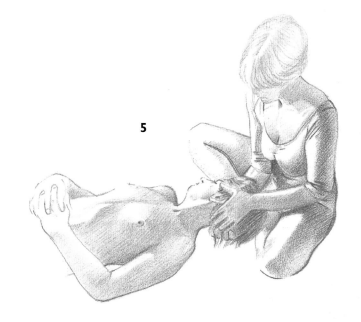

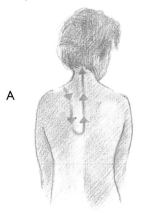

A

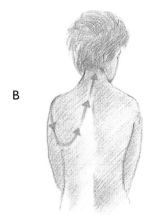

B

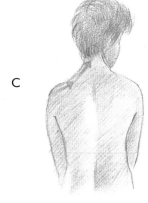

C

A Begin with your hands on the upper chest, just below the collarbone, fingers pointing inward. Pull your hands outward, then curve them round the shoulder joints and slide them along the tops of the shoulders, until you come to the back of the neck. Push down alongside the spine, then pull your curved fingers very slowly up the groove at the side of the spine and up the back of the neck to the base of the skull. Now circle with your fingers all along this side of the base of the skull, working just under the rim of the bone. Repeat once more.

B Begin as before, but when your hand reaches the shoulder joint, curve your fingers round under the shoulder and push down along your partner's side. When you reach the waist, pull diagonally across the shoulder blade, with fingers slightly curved, until you come back to the neck. Then circle along the base of the skull again. Repeat twice more.

C Begin as before, but once your hand has circled the shoulder joint, pull along the top of the shoulders and up the side and back of the neck with your thumb over the front of the shoulder and your fingers behind. The inside edge of the index finger and the web of the thumb should create a taut band. After circling as before at the base of the skull, repeat the stroke. Then leave your partner's head in your hands, ready to work on the scalp.

NECK, HEAD, BACK, AND SHOULDERS

Step 7
Spread your hand over the head and rotate it, moving the scalp against the bone.

Step 8
Rub vigorously all over the scalp with your fingertips.

Step 9
Taking a bunch of hair at a time, pull from the roots and slowly slide your fingers off.

Turn your partner's head to the other side, rest it on your cupped hand and repeat steps 5 to 9 on the other side.

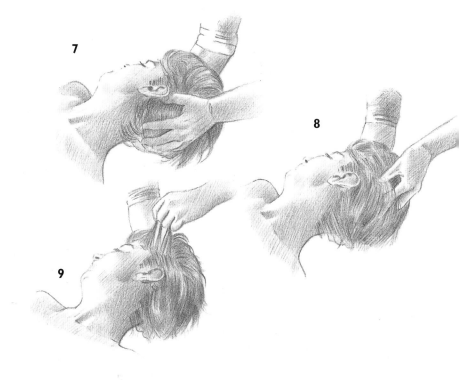

Step 10
Ask your partner to arch her back a little so that you can push your hands as far as possible down her back, placing your palms alongside the spine (A). Now ask your partner to relax on to your arms. Once you feel that she has fully "let go", start to rock your body backward, pulling your hands up the grooves beside the spine (B), up the neck and back of the head (C) and end by "pulling" the hair.

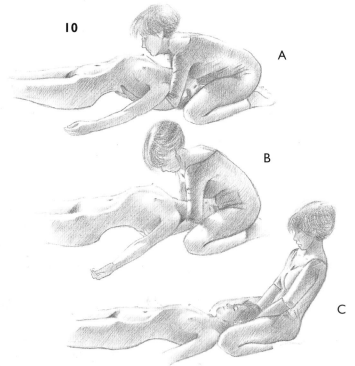

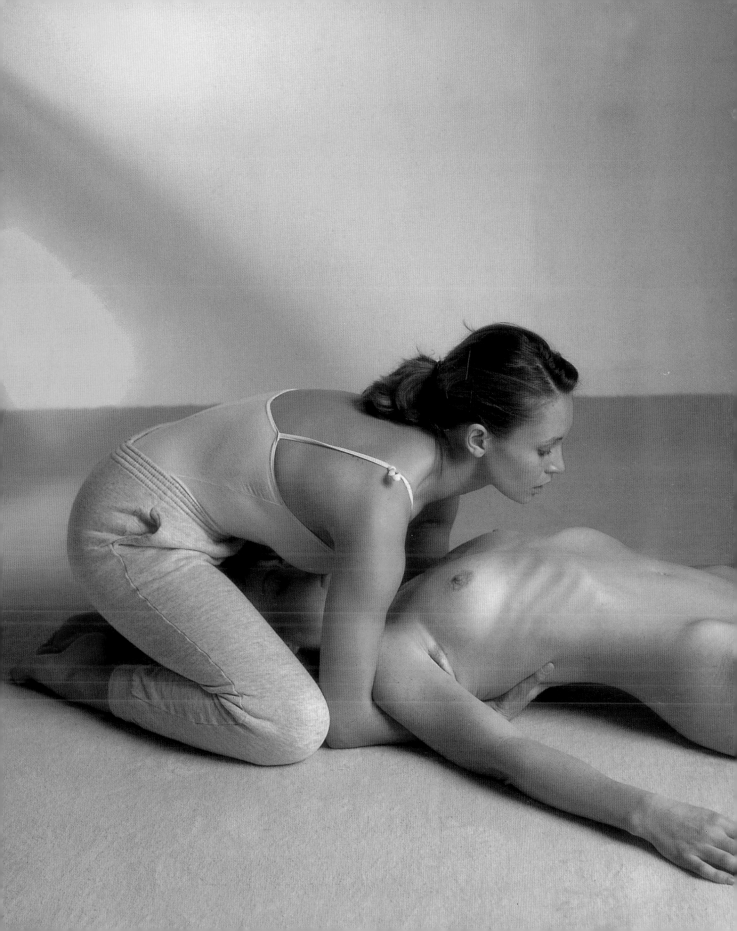

FACE

You may not need to oil your hands to massage the face, as what you already have on your fingers may be enough for this relatively small area. Since many of the strokes on the face are quite small, you need to take care to avoid over-tensing your shoulders. Even the smallest strokes benefit from rocking back and forth from the hips.

If using towels, cover the whole of the front of the body.

Caution*: Before beginning, check whether your partner is wearing contact lenses or has had eye surgery in the past year; if so, do not work over the eyelids.*

Step 1
Still positioned at your partner's head, place your thumbs at the centre of the forehead, just above the brows, anchoring your hands on the sides of the head. Draw your thumbs apart slowly, coming out over the hair and off the sides of the head. Then return your thumbs to the centre, moving them up about 1 cm (0.5 in), and repeat. Cover the whole forehead in this way, up as far as the hairline.

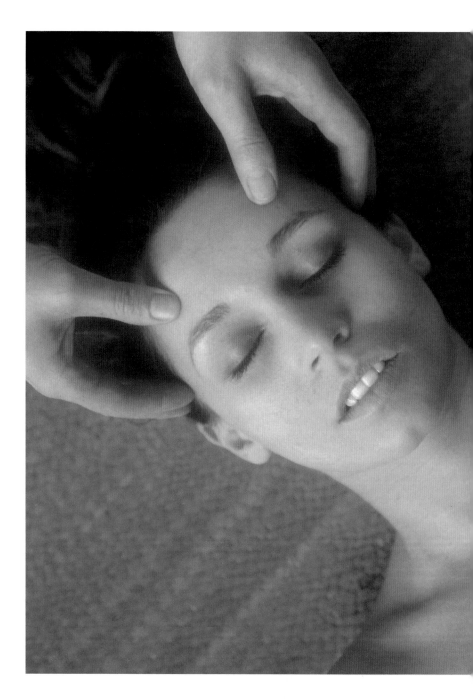

Step 2
Starting at the inner end of the eyebrows, draw your thumbs firmly out to the sides, over the hairline and off the head, smoothing the entire browline. Repeat four times.

Step 3
Draw your thumbs smoothly and gently over the eyelids, from the inner to the outer corners and off the sides of the head. Repeat twice.

Step 4
Stroke down the bridge of the nose from the top to the tip, using alternate thumbs. Then squeeze the tip of the nose gently between your thumb and index finger.

Step 5
Beginning just under the inner corner of the eyes, stroke your thumbs across the cheekbone to the hairline above the ear and off the head. Repeat the stroke, moving your thumbs down 1 cm (0.5 in) each time as you gradually cover the whole face in this way. When working near the nose, be careful not to close the breathing passages.

Caution: *Do not use this stroke on anyone who has had surgery on their sinuses.*

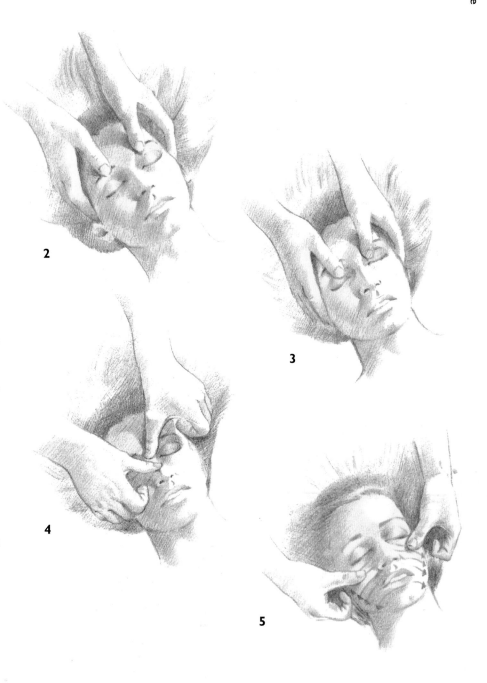

2

3

4

5

FACE

Step 6
Hold the point of the chin between your thumbs and index fingers, then draw your hands slowly apart, squeezing along the whole chin, using a rhythmical "milking" stroke.

Step 7
Hold the rim of the jawbone at the chin, then draw your hands slowly apart, squeezing right along the jawbone as far as the ear lobe. If your partner holds a lot of tension in the hips, it is often helpful to loosen the jaw in this way before working directly on the pelvis.

Step 8
Locate the chewing muscles on each side of the face. Then circle slowly over them with the pads of your fingers.

Step 9
Place the heels of your hands on either side of the nose. Now slowly part your hands, gliding them firmly over the cheeks and out toward the ears.

Step 10
Grasp the ears between your fingers and the heels of your hands and very gently stretch them away from the head. Then squeeze all around them with your fingers and thumbs.

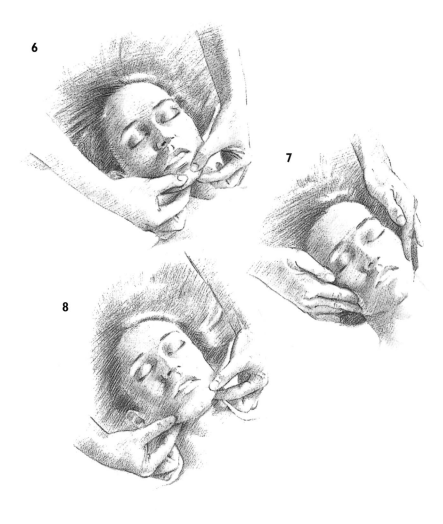

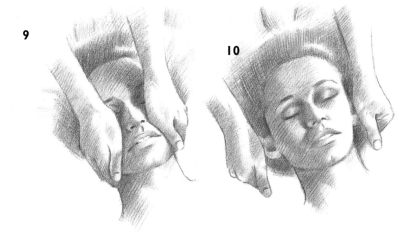

Step 11

Cup your palms over your partner's eyes, with your thumbs on either side of the nose and fingers pointing toward the chin. Remain there for a moment, allowing the eyes to rest within the darkness of your hands (A).

Then begin to slide your hands smoothly down over the face, out across the cheeks and under the ears to the back of the neck (B).

Pull your hands up the neck and, cupping your hands under the back of the head, draw them toward you, coming slowly off the top of the head and then the hair (C).

Repeat the stroke several times, then finish by resting one hand lightly on the forehead and the other on the upper chest to connect head and body.

After a moment or two, softly break contact.

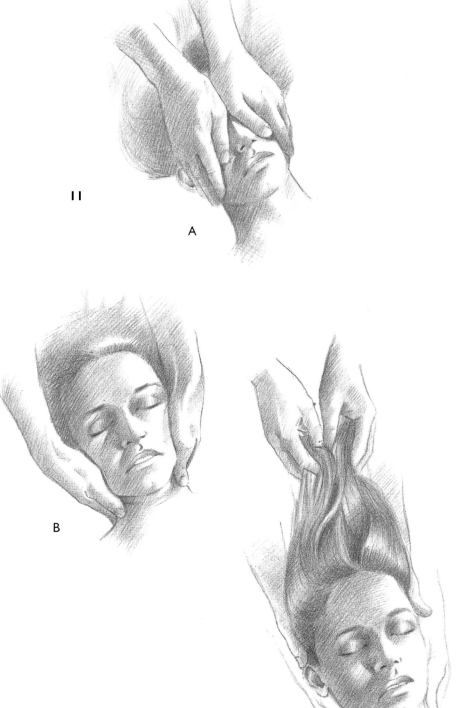

11

A

B

C

ARMS AND HANDS

If using towels, uncover one arm at a time.

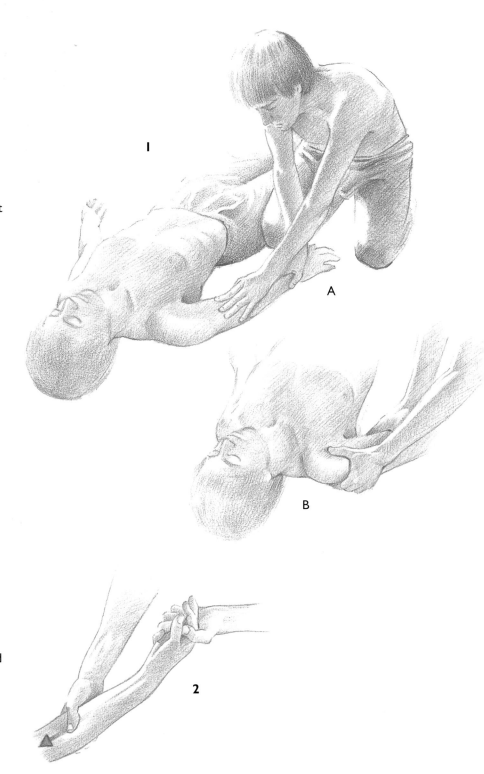

Step 1

Move to your partner's side, level with the hips and facing the head. Start by oiling and warming one of the arms, using the long stroke. Rest your oiled hands on your partner's wrist, fingers pointing up the arm. Now glide your hands up the arm, undulating over the contours (A). Just before you reach the shoulder joint, let your "outside" hand curve over the joint, while your other hand curves down on to the inner arm, just below the armpit (B). Embracing as much of the arm as possible, pull your hands down the arm to the wrist. Enfold your partner's hand in your two palms as you slide them down and off the fingertips. Repeat the whole stroke twice more.

Step 2

Lift your partner's forearm slightly and hold his hand in one of yours. With your other hand hold the wrist between your fingers and thumb, your thumb lying across the inner wrist. Now rock forward as you squeeze down the arm from wrist to elbow. Rock back again and repeat once or twice. This stroke assists the lymphatic flow and the blood's venous return to the heart.

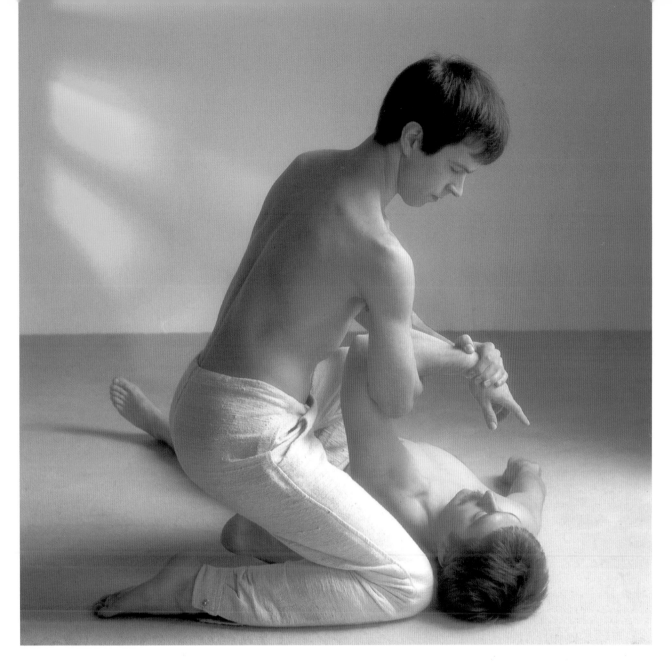

Step 3

Lift your partner's arm and let it bend at the elbow with the hand hanging down on the other side of the neck, so that the upper arm rises vertically. Grasp it near the elbow between both hands and pull down toward the shoulder joint, squeezing firmly. Repeat a couple of times.

3

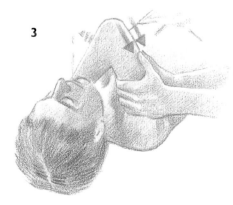

Step 4

Kneeling at your partner's shoulder, link one arm under the elbow joint (your left arm under his right and vice versa, see above), making sure that the crooks of the arms are together. Take hold of your own opposite forearm near the elbow, and with your free hand anchor your partner's wrist. Now lift the arm, stretching the shoulder up off the floor. Let it down gently. Repeat if you wish.

ARMS AND HANDS

Step 5

Take hold of your partner's wrist and lift the arm above the head. Now pull gently on the wrist to give a final stretch to the arm while running your other hand firmly down the side of the ribcage from the armpit, to stretch all the way along the arm and side. Replace the arm by your partner's side.

Step 6

Place one hand on the middle of your partner's upper chest, below the collarbone, the other under the upper back, just below the neck. Sandwiching the body between your hands, draw them slowly toward the shoulder joint, leading with the heels of your hands (A). Repeat this a few times.

The final time that both hands reach the joint, curve them around the top of the arm and work deeply around the joint (B). Seek out the inner structures of bones and joint with the fingers.

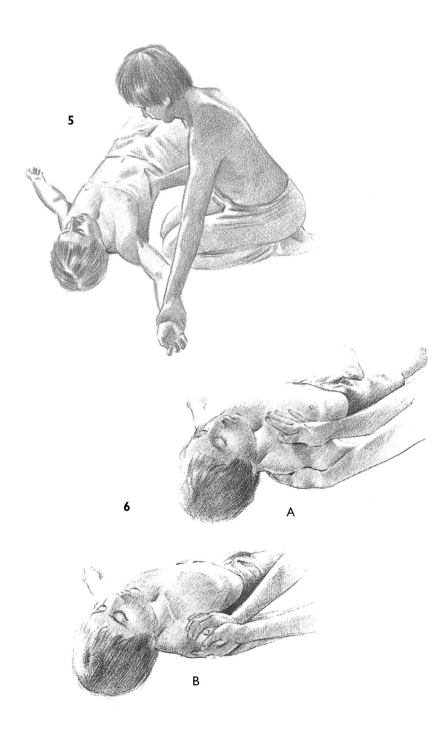

5

6

A

B

56

Step 7

Massage down the arm, kneading and wringing the whole limb until you reach the wrist. Give some attention to the elbow, exploring around the joint with your thumb and fingertips.

Step 8

Lift your partner's forearm, resting the arm on the elbow. Now use your thumbs to work in small circles over the whole wrist area, holding the wrist between your thumbs and fingers.

Step 9

Grasp the hand with your fingers on the palm and the heels of your hands on the back. Now squeeze and stretch the hand open by drawing your fingers away from one another while pressing the heels of your hands down. Repeat once or twice. For the sake of clarity, this illustration is shown from below.

Step 10

Hold your partner's wrist to support the hand. Now use the thumb and index finger of your free hand to work along each of the grooves between the bones of the hand, from the wrist to the web between the fingers.

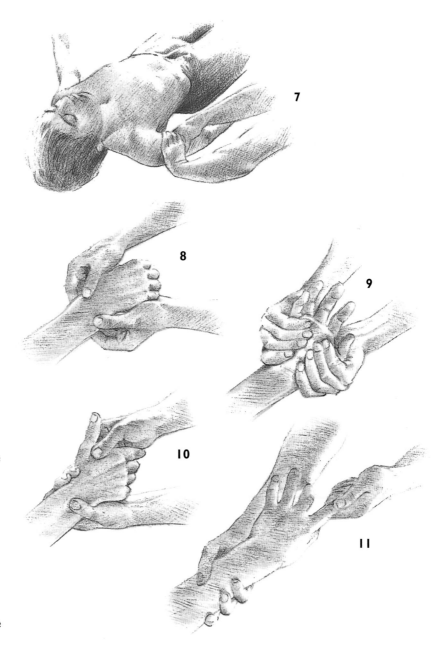

Step 11

Enclose the thumb and each of the fingers in turn in your hand and gently pull them, stretch them, and twist them as you slide your hand down and off the tip.

Now move round to your partner's other side, and repeat steps 1 to 11 on the other arm.

UPPER BODY

If using towels, bare the front of the torso.

Step 1
Position yourself by the top of your partner's head. Oil your partner's torso, starting by resting your hands gently on the middle of the upper chest. Then rock forward from your hips, letting your hands glide slowly down the centre of the torso, allowing them to mould to the forms. On women, take care to avoid the breasts. Just below the navel, let your hands divide and curve out to the sides. Then rock back, pulling your hands back up the body along the sides. Repeat until the torso is oiled.

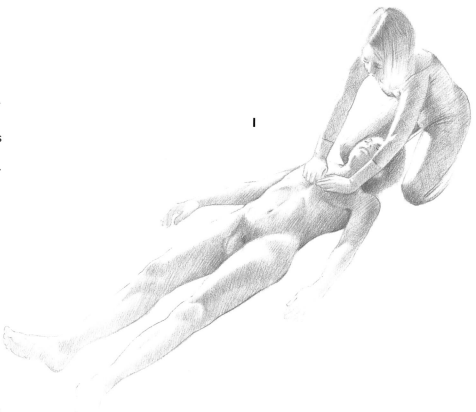

Step 2
Repeat the long stroke from step 1, but when your hands divide below the navel, let them describe large overlapping circles as you travel smoothly back up the sides.

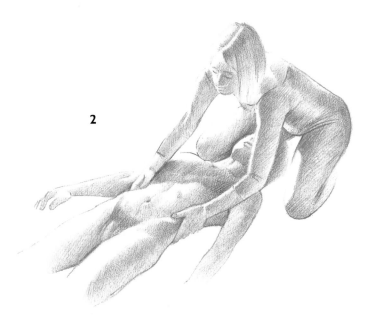

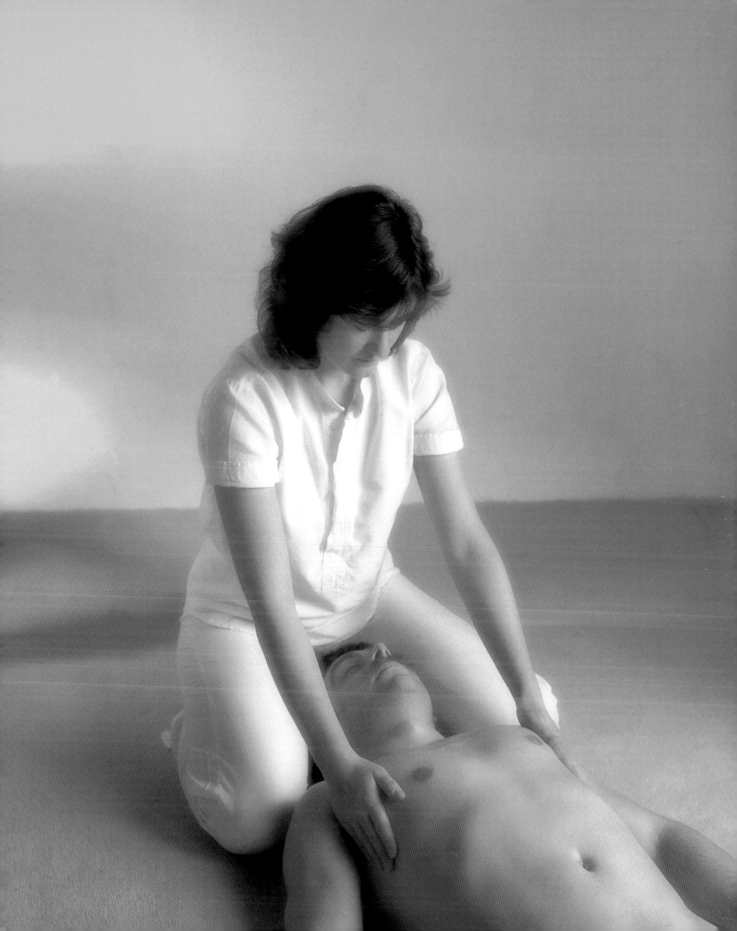

UPPER BODY

Step 3

Place the first two fingers of both hands, pointing toward each other, at the centre of the upper chest in the grooves on either side of the topmost rib (A). Pressing firmly, draw your fingers out to the sides and off the body. Repeat, moving down to the grooves on either side of the rib below. Continue right down the ribcage in this way, as if tracing the rungs of a ladder.

When you reach the bottom of the breastbone, you will find that the ribs no longer start at the centre and you must curve your hands round to work along them (B). Avoid working on the ribs that lie directly under the breast. When you reach the breast, press along the grooves for a short distance only, then move down to the next rib; don't press into the soft tissue of the breasts themselves. Once past the line of the breasts continue the full stroke.

Step 4

Leaning over your partner, use alternate hands to pull up one side of the ribcage from the waist to the armpit. Work around, not directly across, the breasts.

Step 5

Still working on the far side of your partner's body, thoroughly knead the pectoral muscle – the muscle that forms the pit of the arm and supports the breast.

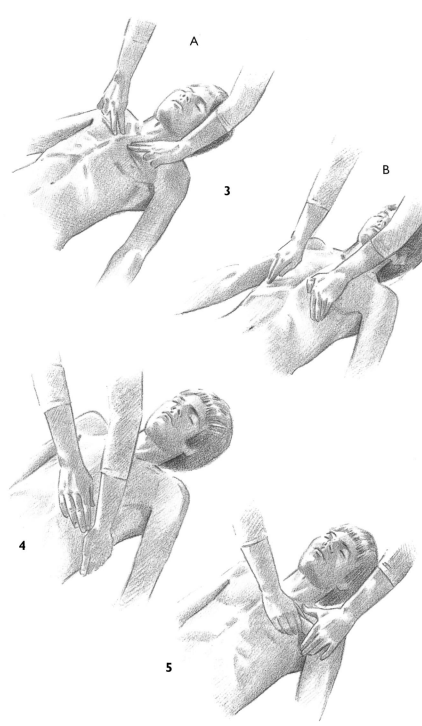

Move round to your partner's other side and repeat steps 4 and 5 on the other side of the body.

Step 6

Still at your partner's side, move so you are level with the abdomen. Let your hands come to rest very gently on the belly and remain there for a moment. Then move both hands clockwise around it, letting them flow over the contours. One hand can complete whole circles, but the other will have to break contact each time the hands cross.

Step 7

With your hands still moving in a clockwise direction, divide your broad circles up into smaller ones, letting your hands spiral round as they travel over the belly.

Step 8

Ask your partner to breathe slowly and deeply. Facing the head, rest your hands on the belly, fingers pointing up the body. As your partner inhales and the chest rises, slide your hands up the centre of the torso (A). As your partner exhales and the chest contracts, circle your hands round the shoulders and pull down the sides of the torso (B). Follow your partner's breath with your hands – not vice versa. Bring your hands back to the belly and repeat from the beginning, two or three times. When you pull your hands down the sides for the last time, continue down over the hips and off the feet.

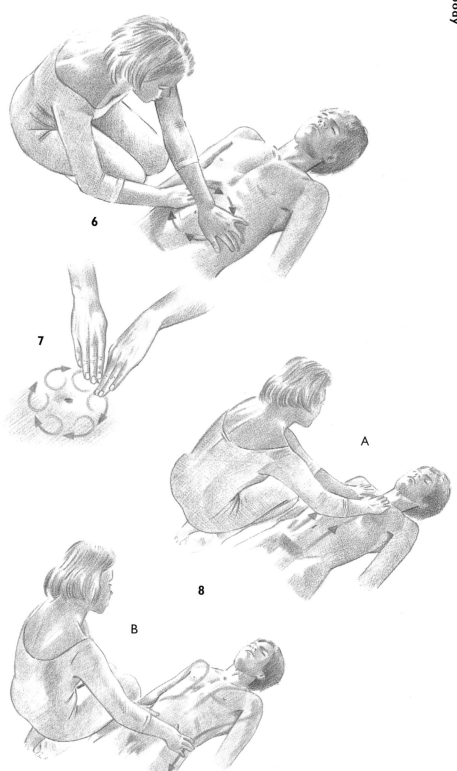

6

7

A

8

B

FRONT OF LEGS AND FEET

*If using towels, cover the whole body,
uncovering one leg at a time.*

Step 1

Position yourself between your
partner's feet. Begin to oil the leg by
resting your hands on the ankle,
fingers pointing up the leg. Then let
them glide slowly up the leg, as you
rock your body forward. When you
near the top, curve your inner hand
down the inside thigh while your
other hand circles around the hip
joint. Take care to respect your
partner's privacy when working on
the inner thigh. Then rock backward,
gliding both hands lightly down the
sides of the leg and off the feet.
Repeat until the leg is oiled.

Step 2

Cup one hand around your
partner's heel, the other across
the top of the foot. Lean back until
your arms are taut, like ropes. Now
raise the foot a little and lean back
from your pelvis, shaking the leg
slightly as you pull. Release slowly,
then repeat.

Caution: *If your partner has varicose
veins, avoid all but gentle strokes up
the leg, as deep massage may
aggravate the condition. Work on either
side of the veins and do not stroke
down the leg at all.*

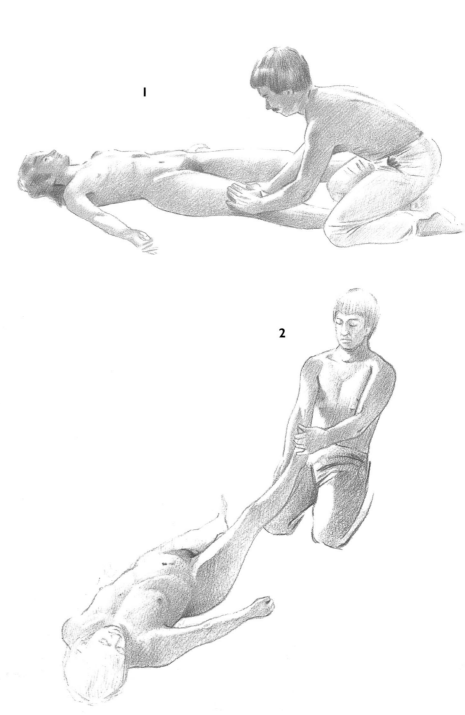

1

2

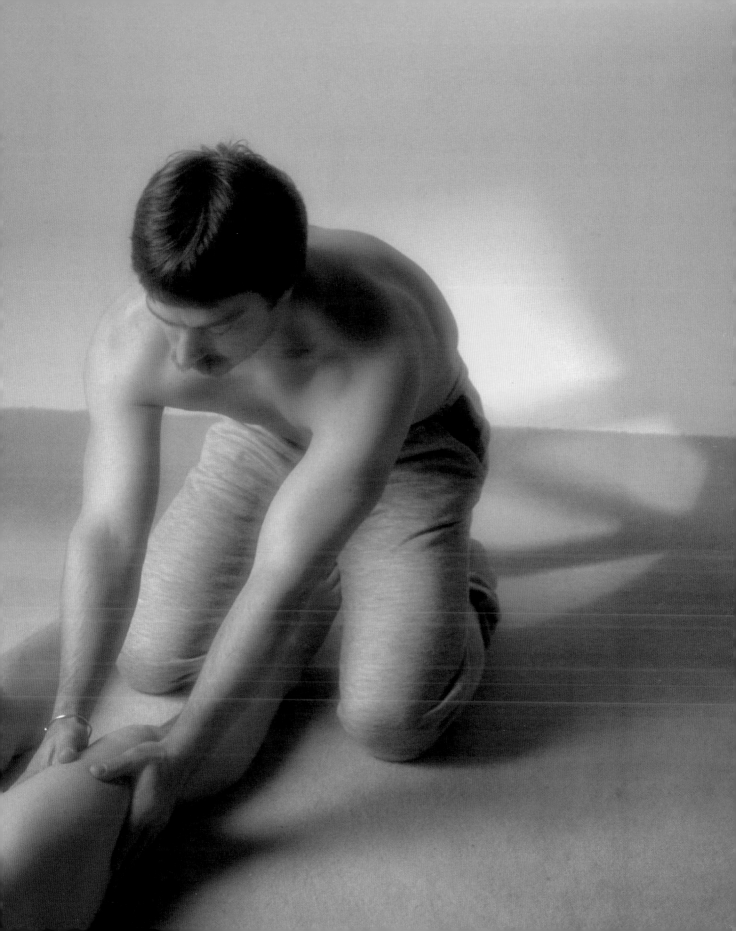

FRONT OF LEGS AND FEET

Step 3

Use the "V" between your thumbs
and fingers to press firmly along
the muscles on either side of the
shinbone. Avoid putting direct
pressure on the shinbone, which
can be painful for the receiver. Move
your hands alternately, letting one
follow the other rhythmically from
ankle to knee. Repeat several times.

Step 4

Overlap your thumbs just above
the kneecap, anchoring your fingers
on either side of the knee.
Simultaneously draw your thumbs
away from each other to circle
around the bone from opposite
directions, letting them cross above
and below the kneecap. Circle
several times.

Step 5

Use both hands alternately to
push up the thigh from the knee
to the top of the leg. Let your
thumbs circle up and outward
as you move gradually up the leg.
Repeat several times.

Step 6

Position yourself facing your
partner's hip. Place both your
thumbs on the side of the buttock
nearest you, 6 cm (3 in) below the
rim of the pelvis. Now knead
around the joint, pushing in deeply
with alternate thumbs. Use the rest
of your hands to "anchor" you.

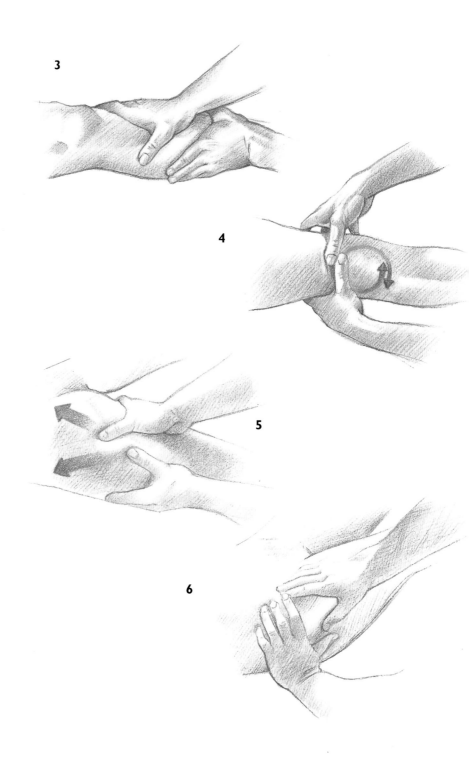

3

4

5

6

Step 7

Starting at the top of the leg, gather and squeeze large bunches of flesh down the thigh, then wring or pull along it. Work around the knee with your fingers, then continue down the lower leg, squeezing alongside the shinbone to the ankle joint. As you work down the leg, you will need to move. When working on a massage table it is easy to move smoothly; but if working on the floor you will probably have to break contact gently, change position, then continue.

Step 8

Move to sit or stand facing the foot you are working on. Clasp the foot with your fingers under the sole and your thumbs alongside one another on the top. Squeezing the foot firmly, draw the lengths of your thumbs away from each other, opening the foot and stretching the bones apart.

Step 9

Sandwich the foot between your hands, fingers pointing up the leg. Draw your hands slowly toward you and slide gently off the toes. Repeat a few times.

Repeat steps 1 to 9 on the other leg.

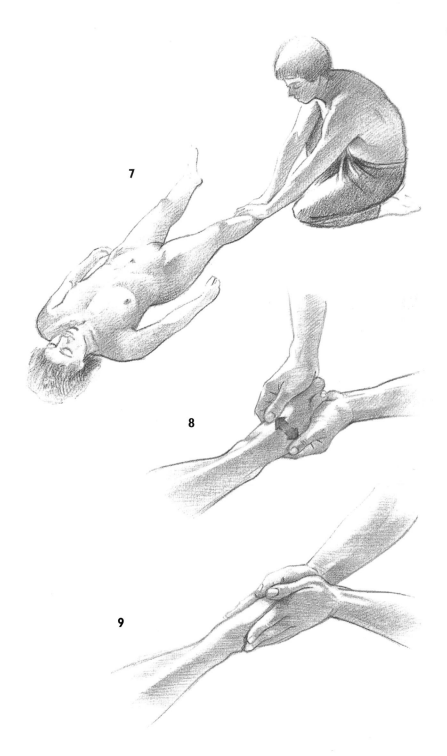

CONNECTING

If using towels, cover the whole body and make the strokes in step 1 lightly over the towels.

Step 1

Having worked on each part of the body in turn, you now need to "connect" the various parts and give your partner a sense of wholeness.

Position yourself by your partner's side, at hip level, so that you can reach both ends of the body at once. Rest the fingertips of both hands side by side on the forehead, then move lightly up over the top of the head, down the back of the neck, down the arms, and off the fingertips. Repeat, but when you reach the base of the neck, come round to the front and down the torso. At the navel, separate your hands and come down the legs and off the toes.

Step 2

Rest one hand lightly on your partner's forehead and the other on her abdomen. Sit quietly for a moment, before breaking contact and gently releasing both hands together. If you started the massage treatment by making an energy connection, you should break the connection now (see page 31).

Cover your partner with a warmed towel. Leave her to rest for a while. You may wish to use the clearing visualization on page 31 to clear your energy and the energy of the space.

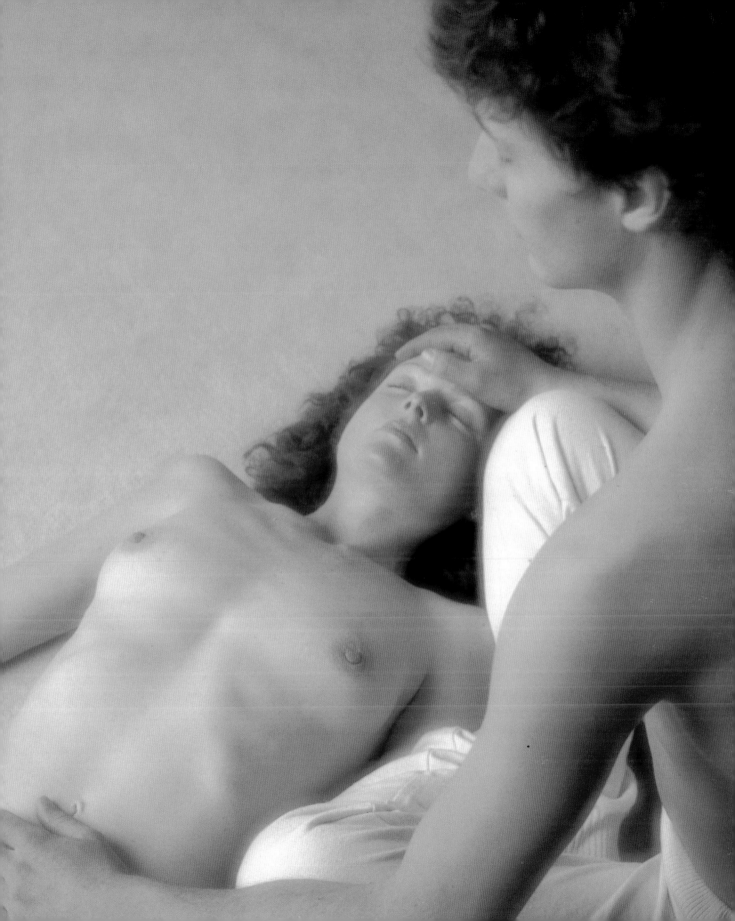

CHAPTER 3

CHINESE MASSAGE

Chinese massage uses manipulation on specific acupoints and Channels to remove Qi–blood stagnation, open the Channels, and balance Yin and Yang energies, thus promoting good health and wellbeing. Care and sensitivity, a little time and energy, a willing pair of hands and knowledge of some basic massage manipulations are all you need to begin.

Your massage strokes should be even and reasonably forceful, so that they are deep and thorough. Your movements should always be continuous, elastic, and above all rhythmic. Keep your hands and arms relaxed as you perform the strokes, increasing the pressure by "leaning in" with your body weight. Be guided by your partner on how much pressure to use. As a rule, you should start the sequence with gentle pressure, increase to stronger pressure for the middle of the sequence, and then end the sequence with gentle pressure again.

The complete massage treatment in this chapter begins with the receiver sitting in a firm, upright chair for work on the head, neck, shoulders, and arms. For the rest of the massage, on the abdomen and front of legs, and then the back and back of legs, the receiver needs to be lying down. The receiver can be either clothed or naked during the massage, as long as the area being treated is bare. Always respect your partner's need for privacy. In the lying-down positions you may wish to use towels to cover the parts of the body you are not working on.

The acupoints to treat are shown on the diagrams throughout the sequence. They are also illustrated in the charts on pages 242–5, with descriptions of how to find them. Remember that they exist in symmetrical pairs on each side of the body, except for points on the Ren and Du Channels, which are on the midline of the body.

Before starting the massage, familiarize yourself with the basic strokes described on pages 16–17. Prepare the room and yourself, following the guidelines on pages 28–30. Ask your partner to sit comfortably in a chair, and position yourself so that you can exert your force effectively. Begin the massage by centring yourself (page 30). You may also wish to use the cleansing visualization (page 30), or make the energy connection between you (see page 31).

Caution: *See page 5 for a full list of cautions and contraindications for massage.*

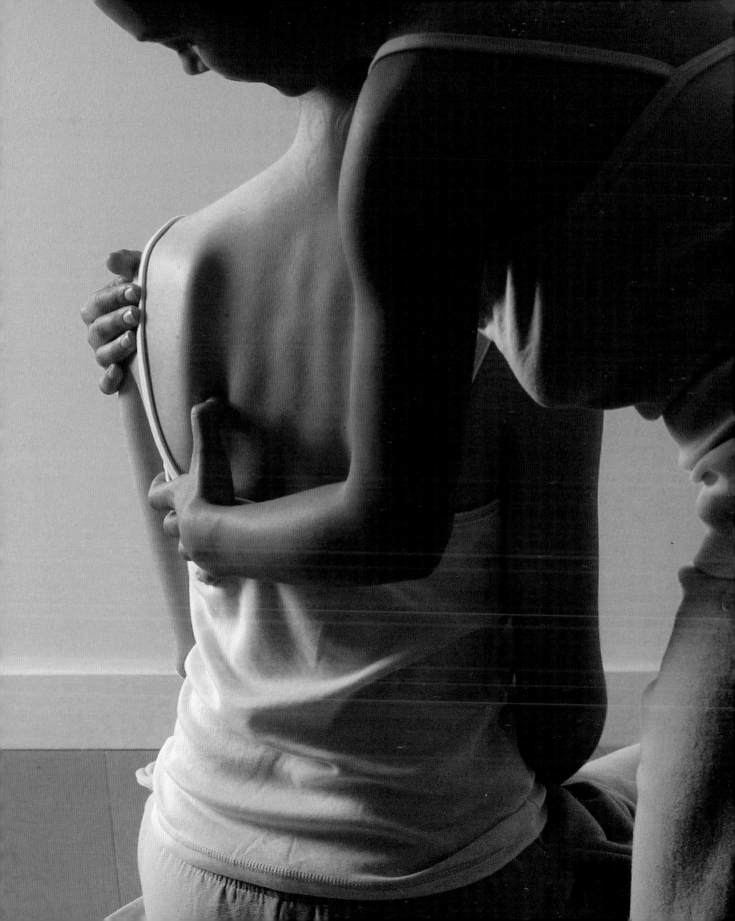

HEAD, NECK, AND SHOULDERS

For this part of the sequence, the receiver should be sitting comfortably in an upright chair.

Step 1

Squeeze and knead both B2 acupoints on the inner end of each eyebrow. Massage the points with your thumb and middle finger, and repeat 20 times.

Press the extra point Yintang (between the eyebrows) 20 to 30 times with your thumb. Then press the acupoints Du23, Du20, Du16, and Du14, 20 to 30 times each in succession.

Step 2

Wipe the eyebrows from the inner to the outer ends with your middle fingers. Apply smooth, even strokes, and repeat 10 times.

Step 3

Press and knead each of the following pairs of acupoints 20 to 30 times: extra point Taiyang on the temples, about 2.5 cm (1 in) beyond the eye socket on a line from the eye to the top of the ear, St8, GB8, and GB20.

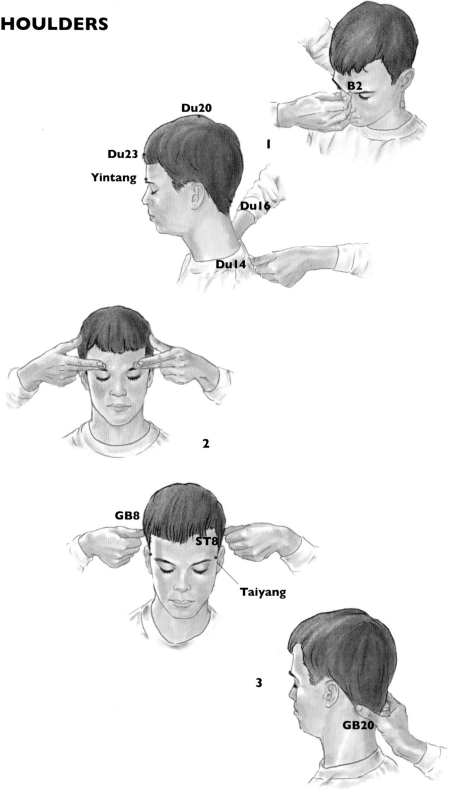

Step 4

Press and knead both St1, both LI20, both SI19, and both St6 acupoints. Massage each pair 20 to 30 times with your thumbs.

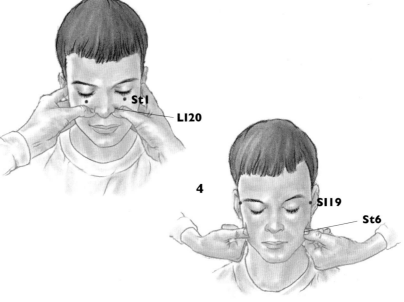

Step 5

Pinch down the outside of both ears from top to bottom, 10 times.

Facing your partner, press your palms over the ears and hold for a minute or two. Keeping your palms on the ears, clench your fists loosely and percuss lightly across the back of the head with the tips of your middle fingers. Keep your wrists relaxed and the percussing action rhythmic and elastic. Repeat 20 times.

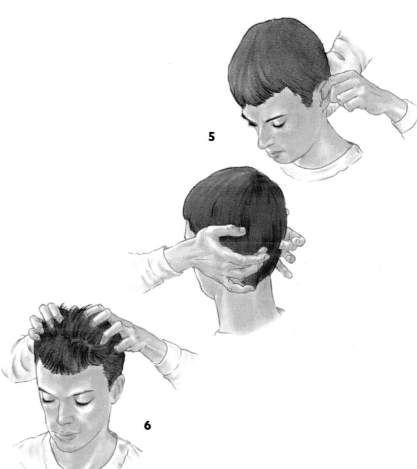

Step 6

Using the tips of your fingers, comb the scalp. Start at the hairline on the forehead and comb to the back of the head. Repeat 20 times.

HEAD, NECK, AND SHOULDERS

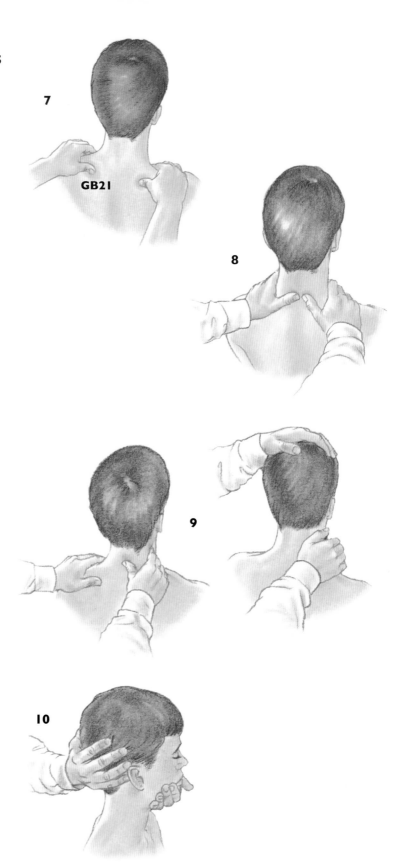

Step 7
Squeeze acupoint GB21 on both shoulders 20 times.

Caution: *Do not massage this point on anyone who is pregnant.*

Step 8
With your palms, rub the neck and the upper back area to encourage your partner to relax.

Step 9
Press and knead up the side of the neck with the heel of your hand. Then squeeze and rub the neck and shoulder muscles, until the muscles feel soft and warm. Repeat on the other side of the neck.

Step 10
Support the head by holding it under the chin and at the back of the head. Raise the head slightly, then slowly and gently turn it from side to side several times.

ARMS AND HANDS

Work through steps 1 to 13 of this part of the sequence on the right arm. Then repeat on the left arm.

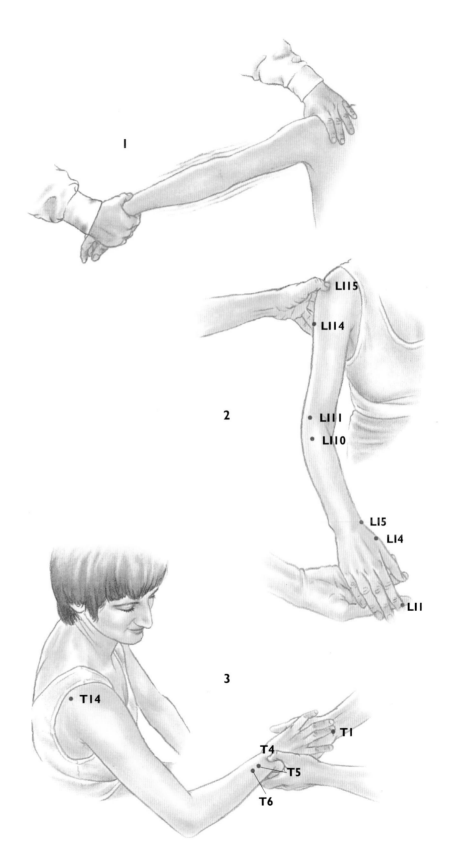

Step 1
Support the right arm at the shoulder and wrist. Ask your partner to relax the arm, then hold the wrist firmly and gently shake the arm up and down, as if it were a rope, 10 times. Keep the movements small and do not let the arm twist. Repeat on the left arm 10 times.

Caution: *Do not massage LI4 on anyone who is pregnant.*

Step 2
Work down the Large Intestine Channel on the arm, pressing the following acupoints one by one, 20 to 30 times with your thumb: LI15, LI14, LI11, LI10, LI5, LI4, and LI1.

Step 3
Using your thumb, press the following acupoints on the Triple Warmer Channel 20 to 30 times each: T14, T6, T5, T4, and T1.

ARMS AND HANDS

Step 4
In sequence, press acupoints SI11, SI9, SI8, SI3, and SI1 on the Small Intestine Channel 20 to 30 times with your thumb.

Step 5
Open the Lung Channel by pressing acupoints Lu5, Lu7, Lu9, Lu10, and Lu11 with your thumb, one by one, 20 to 30 times each.

Step 6
With your thumb, press P3, P6, P8, and P9 acupoints on the Pericardium Channel, 20 to 30 times each, in succession.

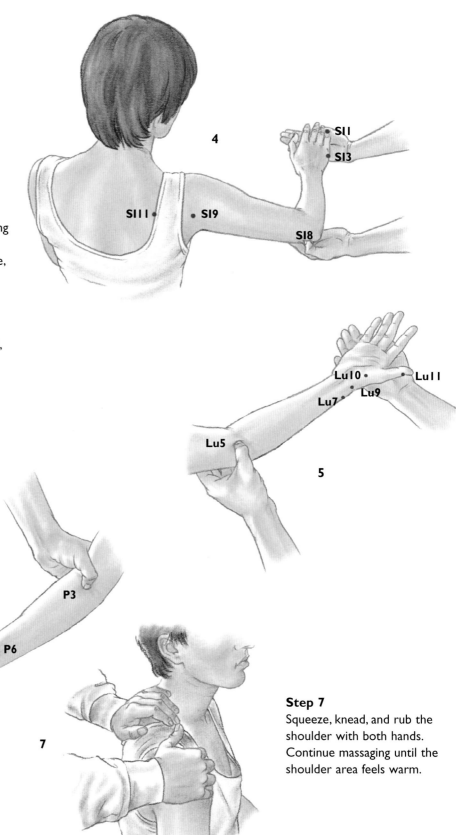

Step 7
Squeeze, knead, and rub the shoulder with both hands. Continue massaging until the shoulder area feels warm.

Step 8

Hold the arm between your palms and twist it by moving your palms back and forth in opposite directions.

Next support your partner's arm at the shoulder and wrist, and then shake the arm up and down gently, as in step 1 on page 73.

Step 9

Still holding the arm at the shoulder and the wrist, circle it clockwise 10 times, gradually enlarging the circle each time. Then circle the arm in an anticlockwise direction 10 times, again increasing the size of the circle each time.

Step 10

Hold your partner's arm out to one side, supporting it at the wrist. Rub the extended arm and hand with your palm. Continue rubbing until the arm feels warm to your partner.

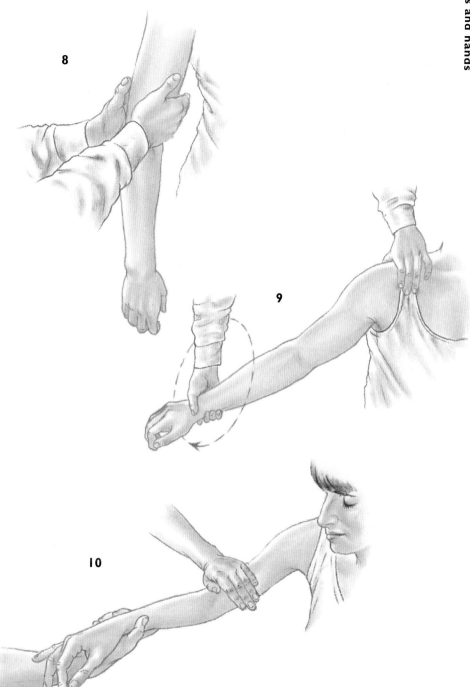

ARMS AND HANDS

Step 11

Support your partner's hand at the wrist, palm upward. Then, with your thumb, press each fingertip in turn, 20 to 30 times.

Step 12

Support your partner's hand at the wrist, palm downward. Then pinch and twist the sides of each finger 20 to 30 times.

Step 13

Place one hand on your partner's shoulder and hold the wrist firmly with your other hand. Shake the arm gently 10 times.

Repeat steps 1 to 13 on the left arm.

Step 14

Using your thumbs, press acupoint LI4 about 30 times on both hands.

Caution: *Do not massage LI4 on anyone who is pregnant.*

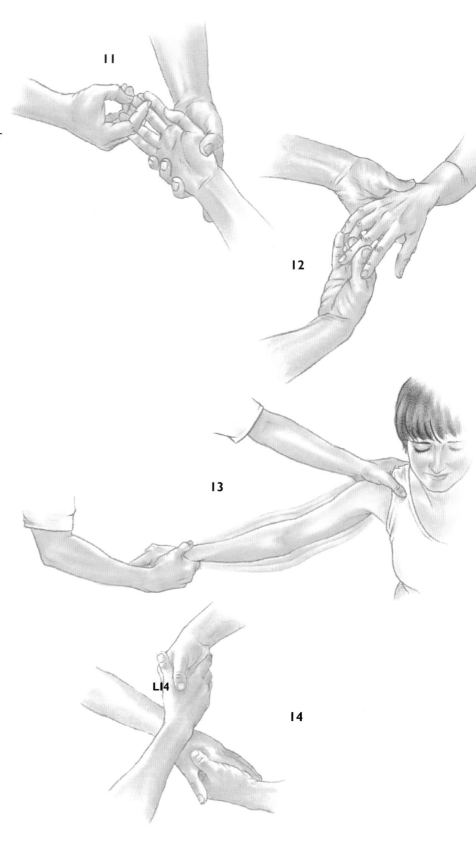

FRONT OF BODY

For this part of the sequence, the receiver should lie face up, either on the floor or on a massage table. Stand or kneel wherever is most comfortable for you to reach the required acupoints easily and apply appropriate pressure.

Step 1

Press Ren17 with the middle finger of your left hand. Keep pressing Ren17 as you work on Ren12, Ren11, Ren9, Ren6, and Ren4 in succession. Use the middle finger of your right hand to press and knead each point 20 to 30 times.

Caution: *Do not massage Ren4 and Ren6 on anyone who is pregnant.*

Step 2

Using your palm, rub 10 clockwise circles around your partner's navel, increasing the size of the circle each time. Then rub 10 anticlockwise circles around the navel. This time, start with a large circle and reduce its size a little each time.

Step 3

Hold both GB26 acupoints, then lift and fold them up over the abdomen. Repeat three times.

Caution: *Do not massage GB26 on anyone who is pregnant.*

Step 4

Press acupoint Ren17 on the midline of the body with your thumb. At the same time, press and knead Liv13 on one side of the body, 20 to 30 times. Then repeat on the other side.

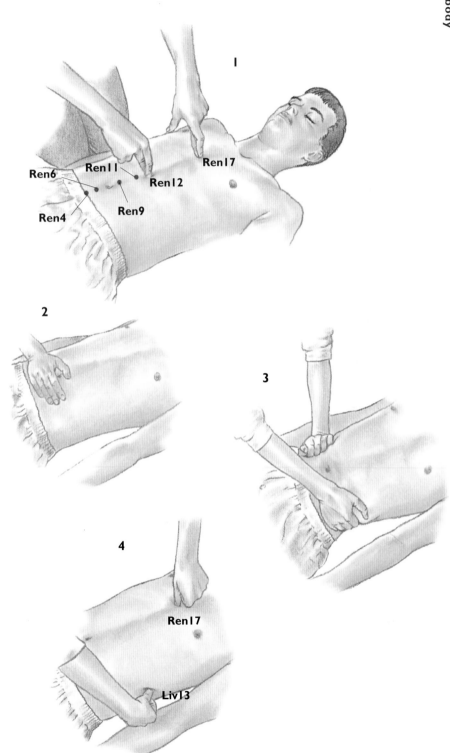

77

FRONT OF BODY

Step 5

Position yourself on your partner's right side and hold acupoint GB26 on the side nearest you, with your left hand. At the same time, press acupoint Sp6 on your partner's right leg with the middle finger of your right hand, 20 to 30 times. Repeat on your partner's left side.

Caution: *Do not massage GB26 or Sp6 on anyone who is pregnant.*

Step 6

Press Ren17 with the thumb of your left hand. At the same time, press both St21 acupoints and then both K18 acupoints with the thumb and middle finger of your right hand. Press each pair 20 to 30 times.

Step 7

Push down the sides of your partner's body with your palms. Repeat three times.

Step 8

Raise your partner's right arm, and press acupoint Lu9 with your left thumb. At the same time, press H1 10 times with your right thumb. Then repeat on the left arm, with hand positions reversed.

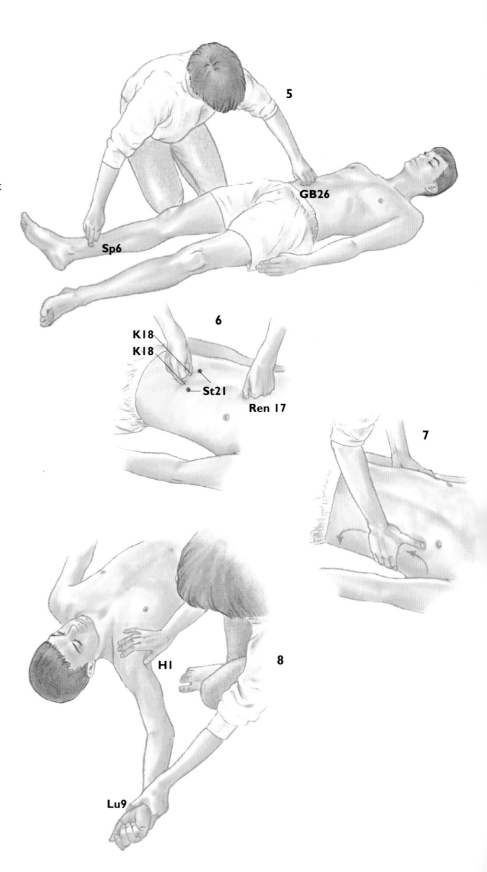

Step 9

Use the fingers of one hand to apply simultaneous pressure to acupoints Ren22, Ren20, and Ren17. Keep your fingers still, and apply constant pressure. At the same time, press Ren14, 20 to 30 times, with the middle finger of your other hand.

Step 10

With the thumb of one hand press Ren14. At the same time, use the fingers of your other hand to press Ren13, Ren12, and Ren10. Press all four acupoints together, 20 to 30 times.

Using the middle finger of one hand press Ren12. At the same time, use the middle finger of your other hand to knead Ren6, Ren4, and Ren3 in succession. Knead each acupoint 20 to 30 times.

Caution: *Do not massage Ren3, Ren4, or Ren6 on anyone who is pregnant.*

Step 11

Using the thumb and middle finger of each hand, knead both St21 and both St25 acupoints simultaneously. Repeat 20 to 30 times.

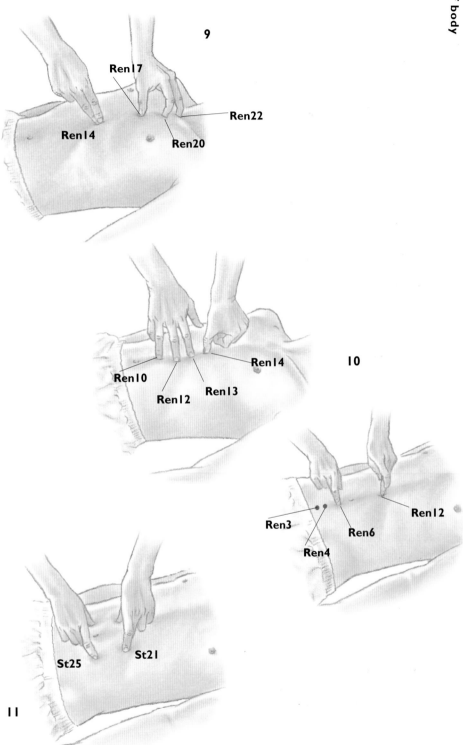

FRONT OF BODY

Step 12

Press Ren15 with your thumb. At the same time, use the thumb and middle finger of your other hand to squeeze acupoints GB34 and Sp9 together on one leg. Squeeze the points 20 to 30 times, then repeat the sequence on the other leg.

Step 13

Press acupoint Lu1 on both sides of your partner's body with your thumbs, 20 to 30 times.

Step 14

Using your thumb, slowly push down the midline of the body along the Ren Channel. Start at Ren22 at the top of the breastbone, and push down to Ren3. Repeat five times.

Caution: *Do not use this step on anyone who is pregnant.*

Step 15

Place your hands, one on top of the other, on your partner's navel. Apply pressure and make a rapid, continuous, quivering action, to penetrate deep down through the skin.

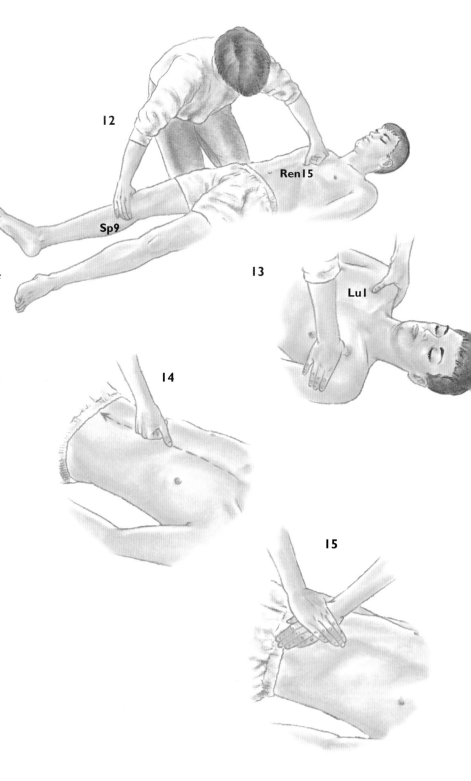

Caution: *Do not use steps 16 and 17 on anyone who is pregnant.*

Step 16
Place the outer side of your hand on the abdomen, with your fingers relaxed and slightly curled. Roll your hand to and fro rhythmically and evenly, applying enough pressure to penetrate the muscle layer. Roll over the abdomen for about one minute.

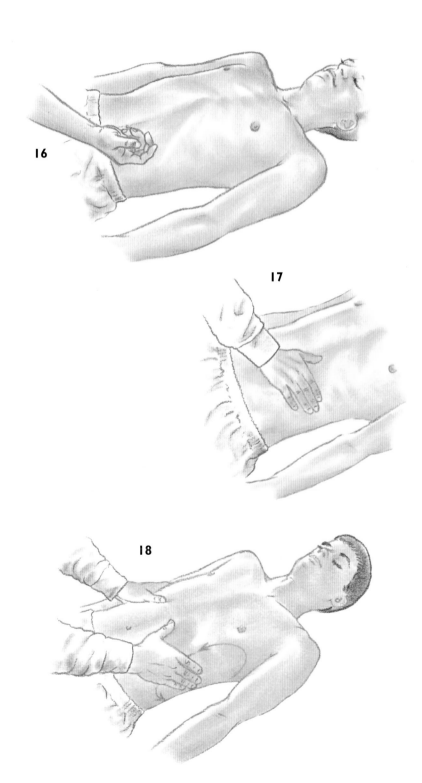

16

17

Step 17
Press and knead the navel with the heel of your hand. Then rub around the navel with your palm until the area feels warm to your partner.

18

Step 18
With your palms, rub down both sides of the abdomen 10 times.

FRONT OF BODY

Caution: *Do not use steps 19 and 20 on anyone who is pregnant.*

Step 19
Press and knead Ren6, Ren4, Ren3, both St29, and both K11 acupoints in succession. Press each point 30 times with the thumb.

Step 20
Squeeze GB26 on both sides of the abdomen. Lift and fold the acupoints up over the abdomen, and then release. Repeat three times.

Step 21
Rub around your partner's navel with your palm. Then repeat step 16 on page 81, rolling the side of your hand backward and forward over the lower abdomen

Step 22
Rub up and down over the upper part of your partner's trunk with your palms. Repeat seven times.

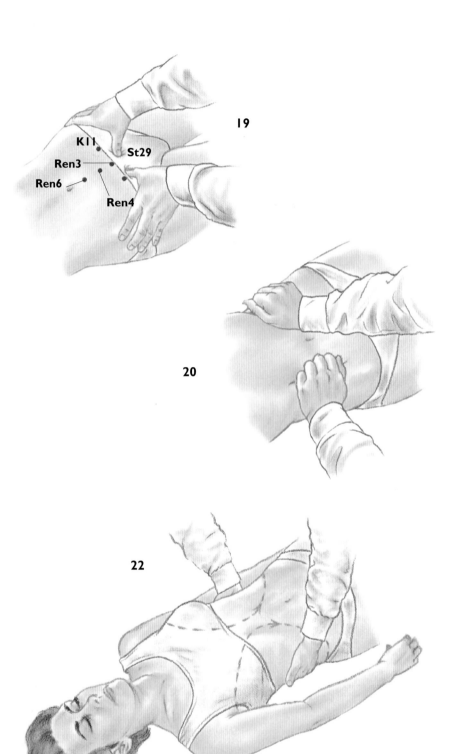

FRONT OF LEGS

Work through steps 1 to 8 of this part
of the sequence on one leg, and then
repeat on the other leg.

Step 1

Press both St30 acupoints with
the heels of your hands for
two minutes.

Using your thumb, press each
of the following acupoints 20 to
30 times in succession: St31, St32,
St34, extra points Xiyan, St36, St40,
and St41.

Step 2

One by one, press the following
points on the Spleen Channel:
Sp12, Sp10, Sp9, Sp6, and Sp4.
Press each point 20 to 30 times
with your thumb.

Caution: Do not massage Sp6 or
Sp12 on anyone who is pregnant.

Step 3

Press acupoints GB30, GB31, GB34,
GB39, and GB40 in succession on
the Gall Bladder Channel. Use your
thumbs, and press each point 20 to
30 times.

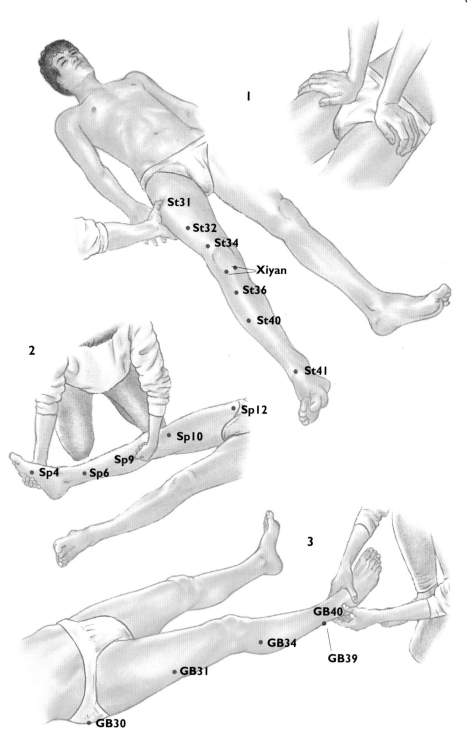

FRONT OF LEGS

Step 4

Knead and rub the knee and the surrounding muscles. Be quite vigorous with this massage, but ensure your partner feels comfortable at all times.

Step 5

Press acupoint GB31, extra point Heding, and acupoints Sp10 and St36 one by one, with your thumb, 30 to 40 times each. Press the extra points Xiyan together 30 to 40 times, then Sp9 and GB34 simultaneously with your thumb and index finger, 30 to 40 times.

Step 6

Support the leg at the knee and ankle and bend and straighten the knee joint. Repeat 20 times.

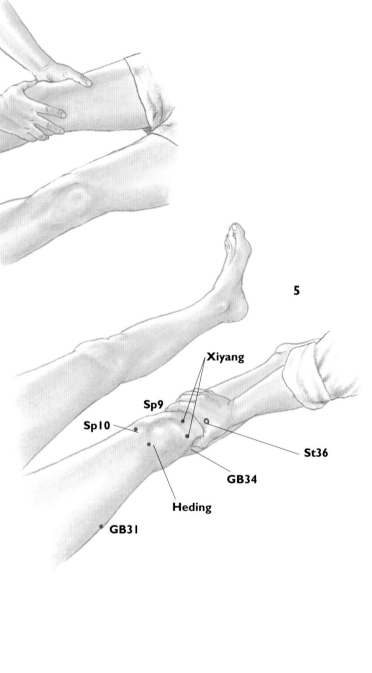

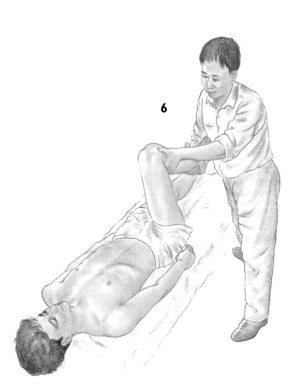

Step 7

Rub up and down over the knee quite vigorously with your palm (A). Then work your way down the leg, kneading the leg muscles with your thumbs (B). Keep rubbing and kneading until the leg feels warm to your partner.

7

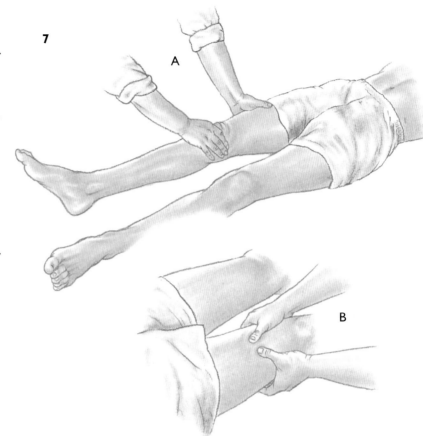

Step 8

Hold the knee between your palms. Move your palms back and forth in opposite directions, moving down the leg to the ankle.

Repeat steps 1 to 8 on the other leg.

8

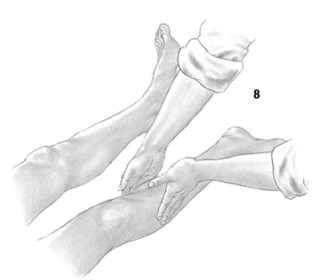

BACK

Ask your partner to roll over on to her front.

Step 1
Position yourself at your partner's head. Rub down the back with your palms using broad, smooth strokes, to relax the back muscles.

Step 2
Press the following pairs of acupoints on both Bladder Channels: B12, B13, B15, B18, B19, B20, B21, B23, B25, and B27. Press each pair 20 to 30 times with your thumbs.

Step 3
Press the group of eight acupoints B31–34 on the Bladder Channel (see page 242) with the heel of your hand on the sacrum, 20 to 30 times. Then move to the other side of your partner's body and repeat.

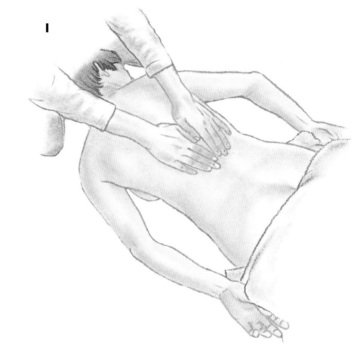

1

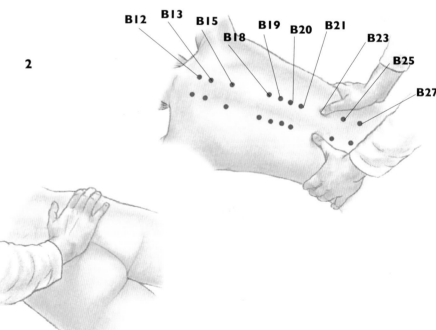

2

B12 B13 B15 B18 B19 B20 B21 B23 B25 B27

3

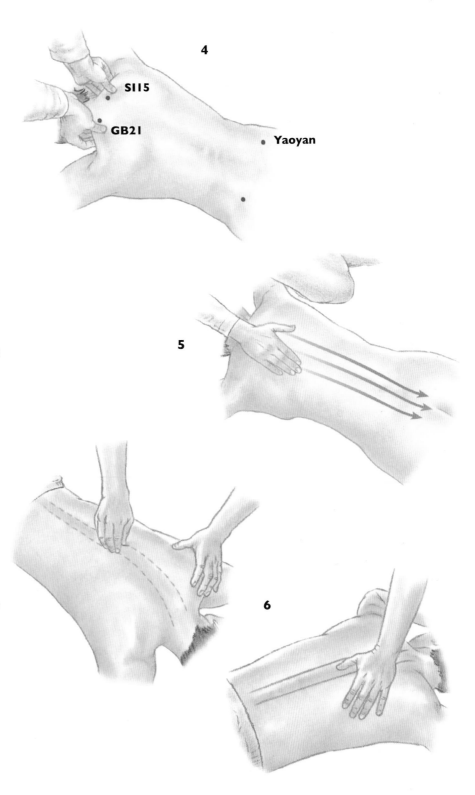

Step 4

Squeeze both GB21 acupoints with your thumbs 20 to 30 times. Press both SI15 acupoints 20 to 30 times, with your thumbs.

Rub both extra points Yaoyan with your palms for one to two minutes.

Caution: *Do not treat GB21 on anyone who is pregnant.*

4

SI15

GB21

Yaoyan

Step 5

Use your palm to press and push down the Du Channel from Du14 to the coccyx. Apply firm pressure, and repeat five times.

Then use your palm to press and push down the Bladder Channel on one side of the spine. Start at B12 and end at B31–34 (see page 242). Repeat five times. Then push down the Bladder Channel on the other side of the spine.

5

Step 6

Work down the back, from top to bottom, pinching the extra points Jiaji (see page 242) either side of the spine. Repeat five times. Then, with your palm, push down the Bladder Channel on one side of the spine again, from top to bottom. Repeat five times. Then push down the Bladder Channel on the other side of the spine five times.

6

BACK

Step 7

Push down the Du Channel with the heel of your hand. Repeat five times. Then push down both Bladder Channels either side of the spine. Repeat five times for each Channel.

Push down and press the spine with the heel of your hand. Then press down the Bladder Channel each side of the spine in turn again. Repeat five times for each Channel.

Step 8

Loosely clench your fist and then percuss rhythmically all over the upper back, using the middle sections of your fingers. Then tap the upper back with your palm for one minute, keeping your wrist relaxed and the tapping rhythmic and elastic.

Step 9

Place your palm on the lower back, apply intense pressure, and make a rapid, continuous quivering action to apply firm pressure deep down through the skin.

Step 10

Percuss the lower back about 20 times, with your fist loosely clenched and using the middle sections of your fingers.

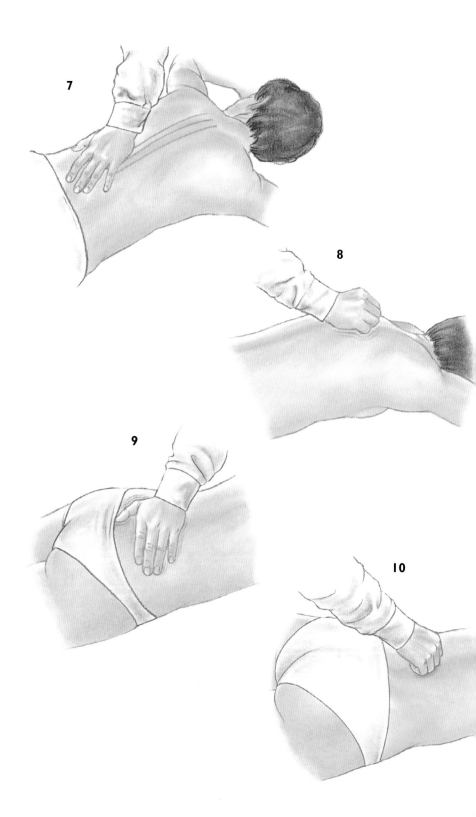

BACK OF LEGS AND FEET

Step 1

Work down both legs simultaneously, pressing the following pairs of acupoints 20 to 30 times with your thumbs: GB30, B37, B40, B57, B60, and K1.

Caution: *Do not massage B60 on anyone who is pregnant, or K1 on anyone with low blood pressure.*

Work through steps 2 to 8 of this part of the sequence on one leg and foot, then repeat on the other leg.

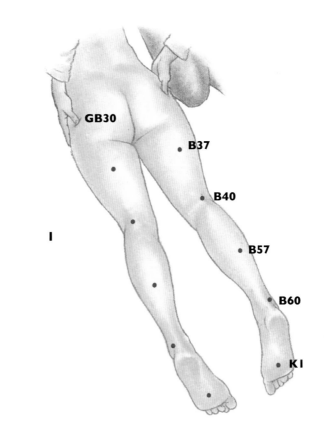

Step 2

Use your thumb to press acupoints K3, K6, and K1 in succession, 20 to 30 times.

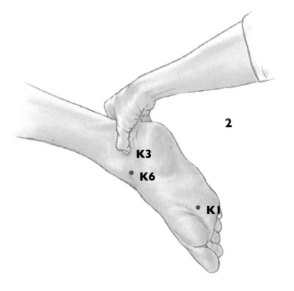

BACK OF LEGS AND FEET

Step 3
Press the lower back with your palm. At the same time, support your partner's ankle from underneath. Raise the leg up then lower it back down, 5 to 10 times.

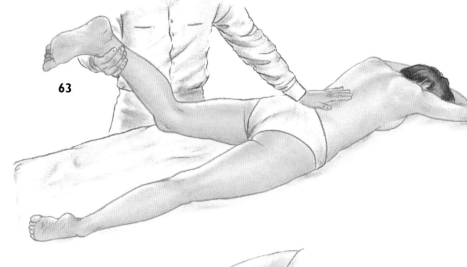

63

Step 4
Form a pincer shape with your hand, and use it to squeeze the muscles down the back the leg.

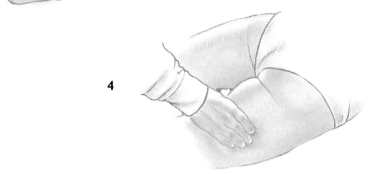

4

Step 5
Squeeze the whole heel area 20 times.

Step 6
Rub acupoint K1 on the sole of the foot, with the heel of your hand. Rub up and down over the point until your partner feels warm there. Then rub over the sole and heel of the foot about 50 times.

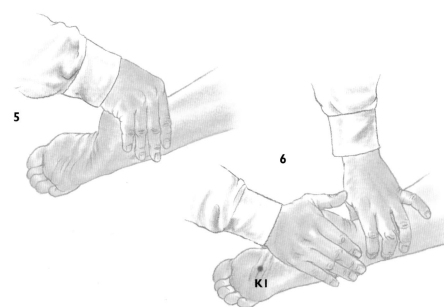

5

6

K1

Step 7

Support your partner's foot by holding the top of the foot with the sole facing you. Starting at the heel and moving along the outer edge of the foot, knead with your thumb quite firmly for a count of five in each position. Move down the edge about two finger widths and repeat until you reach the little toe. Grasp the toe firmly and pull, holding the stretch for a count of three.

Go back to the heel, move one finger width in toward the inner side of the foot, and repeat the sequence. Do this three more times until you have covered the whole foot and pulled each toe in turn.

Step 8

Bend the leg at the knee, so the front of the foot is facing you. Use your middle finger to knead in small circles following four lines between the bones of the foot down toward the toes. Repeat on the other foot.

Repeat steps 2 to 8 on the other leg and foot.

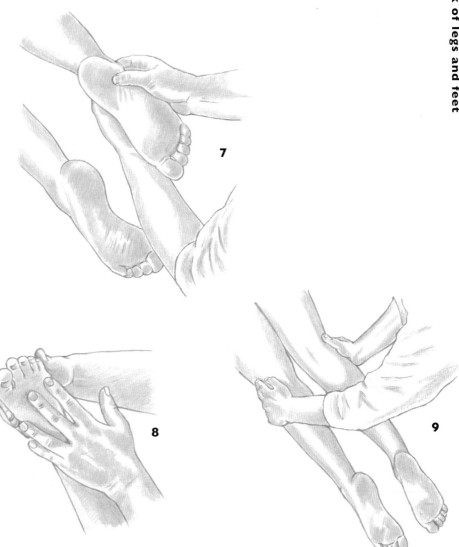

7

8

9

Step 9

This closing sequence follows the rising Yang and descending Yin energies of the body, which helps to smooth out any remaining ripples of unbalanced energy in the back.

Using your whole hand, stroke up the backs of the calves to the knees and down the sides of the legs to the feet three times. On the third sweep continue up the back of the legs to the hips and then down to the knees three times. Then sweep up the back to the shoulders and down the sides to the base of the spine three times.

If you started the massage treatment by making an energy connection, you should break this now (see page 31).

Cover your partner with a warmed towel and leave her to rest for a while. You may wish to use the clearing visualization on page 31 to clear your energy and the energy of the space.

CHAPTER 4

SHIATSU

In shiatsu, the active partner is the "giver' from a practical point of view, but communication through physical contact goes both ways. Your hands work and "listen". You will gain physical support from your partner and respond intuitively to his or her feelings, which means that you give and receive at the same time.

Similarly, when you receive shiatsu massage, you also participate in a two-way process. Allow yourself to feel and respond naturally to any sensations or emotions that arise, and consciously "let go" into the experience. You may feel tense. Sometimes shiatsu can border on the painful, but it should feel like good or helpful pain, never more. Breathe naturally when you feel the pressure and let the tension flow away.

The best shiatsu sessions are often relaxed and quiet, with few words. Both giver and receiver should feed back if there is any discomfort or tension. Either partner may have spontaneous insights during a session – share them, as they may be valuable, but do not let talking interrupt the continuity of the treatment.

Shiatsu is traditionally given with the receiver lying on the floor. Prepare a warm, well ventilated room, arrange a padded area on the floor with a couple of duvets or folded blankets, large enough for your partner to lie down. The padded area should also be large enough for you to work on without slipping off on to the hard floor. You do not require any special equipment to give shiatsu, and no oil is needed. Both giver and receiver should wear loose comfortable clothing. Before you start, familiarize yourself with the basic strokes on page 19. As you become more confident, you can use the techniques on pages 152–3 – "Developing a deep energy connection" and "Working from the Hara" – to enhance your shiatsu. The Hara, or belly, is seen as the seat of Ki or life force.

Begin the sequence with the cleansing visualization and by making the energy connection between you (pages 30–31). This whole-body treatment should take about 30–40 minutes. It begins with the receiver lying face down, with her head turned to one side. Use pillows or folded towels to make her comfortable, and remind her to turn her head to the other side from time to time, to prevent the neck from becoming stiff.

Caution: *See page 5 for a full list of cautions and contraindications for massage.*

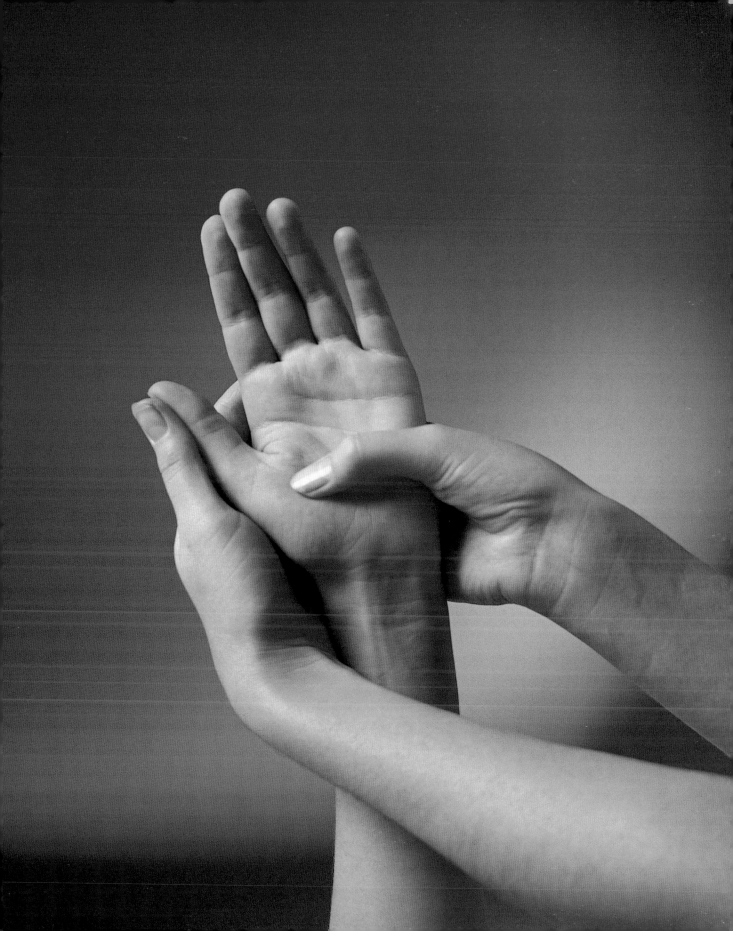

BACK

Kneel next to your partner, if necessary moving her arm a little away from her side to make room for yourself. Breathe into your Hara. Hold your hands at chest level and rub them together briskly and firmly for 30–40 seconds, keeping your shoulders relaxed. This stimulates the flow of Ki in your whole body, and will warm and sensitize your hands for the treatment.

Keep your hands together and your attention focused on how you are feeling for a few moments, before making contact with your partner.

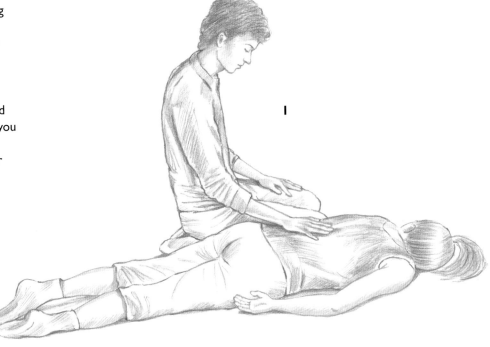

The areas, points, and Meridians to treat are shown in the illustrations for the step-by-step instructions. For more help in locating them, refer to the charts on pages 240–45. To locate body landmarks, such as different areas of the back, see the chart on page 252.

Step I

When you are ready, simply rest your hand on any part of your partner's lumbar (lower back) region. Spend a few moments holding your palm gently in place, giving your partner time to adjust to your contact. Start to focus your attention on the depth and rhythm of your partner's breathing. Visualize your energy connecting with your partner's energy.

Kneel up, and with your hand still in contact, turn to face your partner's body. Place one hand on the sacral region and the other on the thoracic region, on the back of the chest. Lean forward. Let your spine relax, breathe easily, and continue to focus on your partner's breathing for a few minutes.

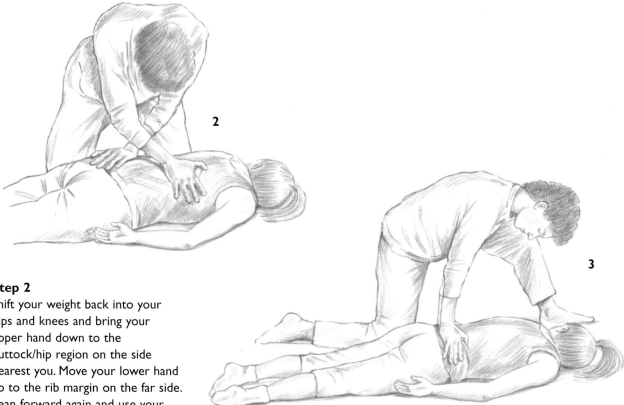

Step 2

Shift your weight back into your hips and knees and bring your upper hand down to the buttock/hip region on the side nearest you. Move your lower hand up to the rib margin on the far side. Lean forward again and use your body weight to create a stretch between your hands. Ask your partner to exhale as you do this.

Hold for a moment, then ease back slightly and bring your hands, one at a time, across to the corresponding opposite positions and repeat the stretch. Repeat both stretches once more, then move round to your partner's other side and repeat twice there.

Step 3

Turn to face your partner's head, then place your hands between the shoulder blades, fingers pointing outward away from each other and the heels of your hands about 2.5 cm (1 in) away from each side of the spine. Move your Hara forward, and lean on to your partner's back, applying pressure. Now ease back and move your hands down, one at a time. When they are level, lean forward again to apply perpendicular pressure.

As you approach the lower spine, move your foot out (see above) to work from a wider base. Sink your weight back, with your arms perpendicular to the lower back and sacro-lumbar region. Lean into the position. Now bring your foot closer to finish with perpendicular pressure on the sacrum. Try to keep these leg movements smooth: your partner will give you the stability you need.

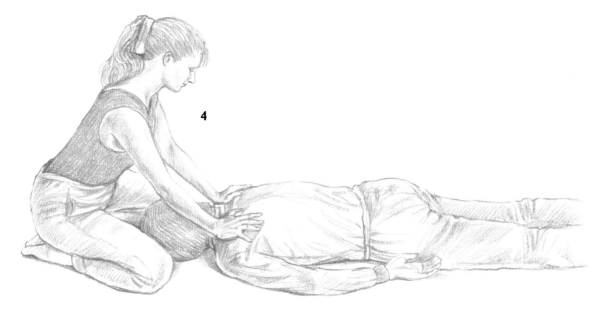

Step 4
Sit, knees apart, at your partner's head. Put a pillow under the chest for greater comfort, especially if your partner's neck is stiff. Relax and lean with your hands over the upper shoulder blade area. Allow a moment to tune in to your partner's condition.

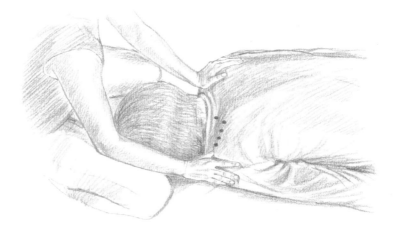

Step 5
Thumb along the SI Meridian from the base of the neck to the shoulder extremity twice each side. Place your support hand on the opposite shoulder. The line runs across the top of the shoulder blade to the hollow point at the end. The Meridian also runs down on to the shoulder blade.

Step 6

Lean with the outside of your hand into the Small Intestine Meridian in the muscly area between the shoulder and the bone of the arm. Then repeat on the other side of the body.

Step 7

Palm the area between the shoulder blades, each side of the spine, using one hand at a time or both together. Then thumb along the inner line of the Bladder Meridian – the ridge of the muscles about 4 cm (1.5 in) from the midline. Work down as far the tip of the shoulder blades, then repeat along the outer line of the Meridian 7.5 cm (3 in) from the midline. Bring your weight forward as you work down.

Step 8

Move to your partner's side, remaining in contact as you do so. Move the arm out a little and on to its edge to bring the little finger uppermost. Palm the arm from the shoulder down to the wrist. Relax your fingers around the arm and steady it with a gentle grip as you explore its contours. Gripping the arm with your thumb on one side and your fingers on the other, make a small rolling motion to apply pressure through the knuckle at the base of the forefinger. This is called the "dragon's mouth" technique. Move up along the arm in this way.

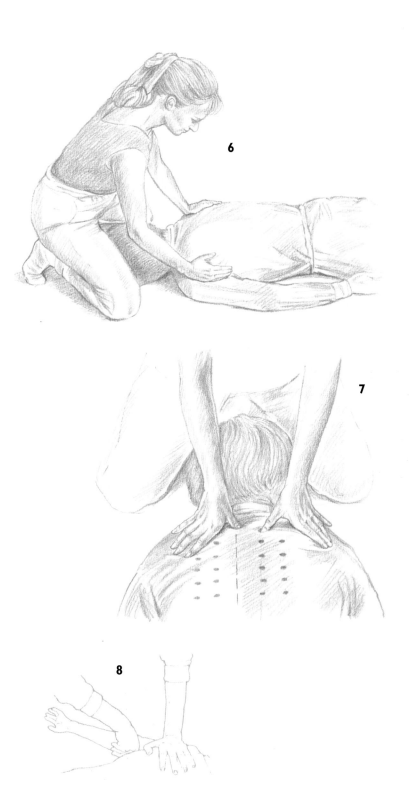

BACK

Step 9

Begin thumbing the SI Meridian at SI8, between the elbow's bony point and the rounded tip of bone on the inside of the joint (A). Then move to the outer edge of the forearm and thumb down to the wrist. After the prominent bone at the wrist, follow the Meridian along the outer edge of the hand, finishing at the little finger (B).

Step 10

Kneel beside your partner and place your support hand on the back between the shoulder blades. Turn your partner's hand so the palm is facing up to expose the inner aspect of the arm, where the Heart Meridian runs.

Gently grasp the upper arm near the armpit and allow your thumb to rest over the bone along the inner border of the biceps muscle. Lean with your emphasis on the thumb side and palm toward the elbow. Then palm the forearm to the wrist. Repeat with a more penetrating angle of the thumb.

Thumb the point H7 "Mind Door" at the wrist crease. This point is well known for its calming but supportive effect on heart and mind. Then thumb along the outside of the palm to the little finger, finishing by gently squeezing along both sides of the finger to the tip.

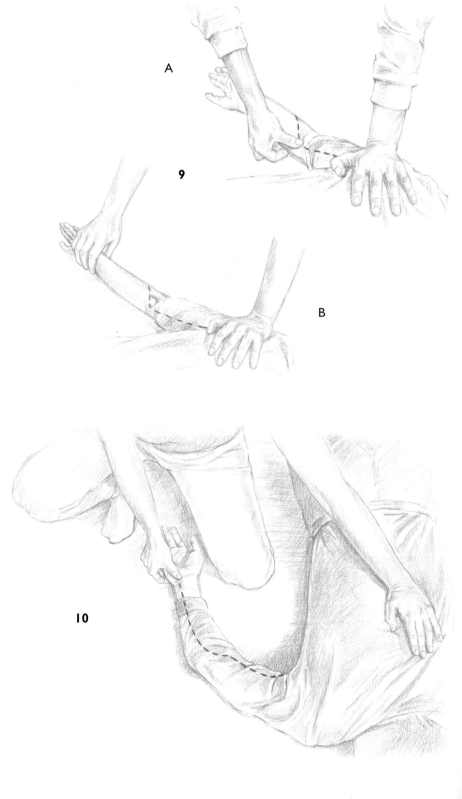

A

9

B

10

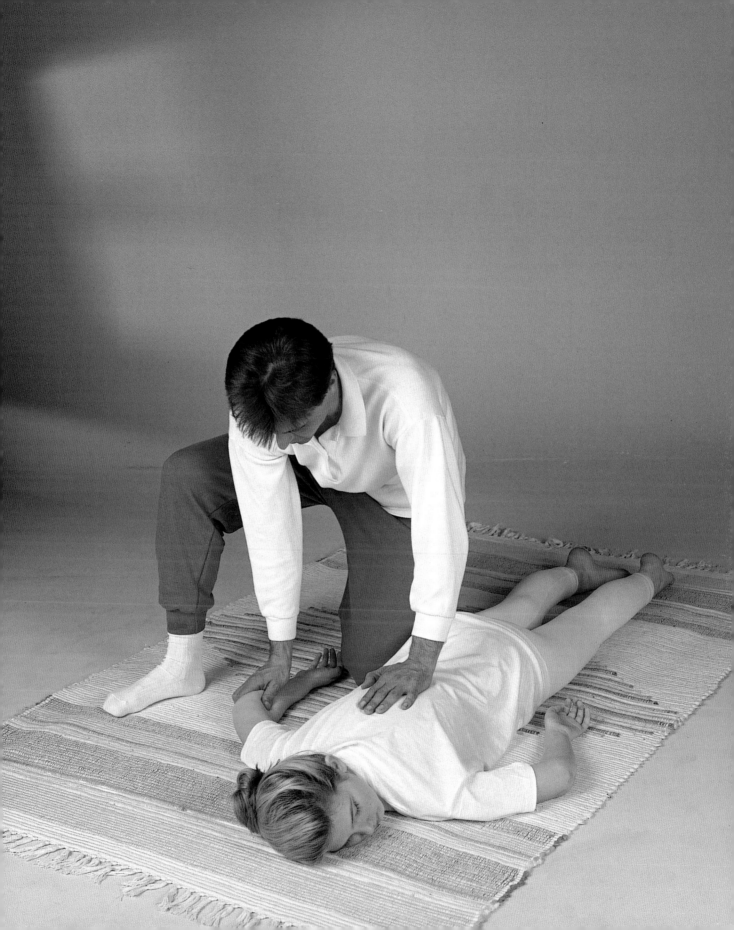

BACK

Step 11

Pick up your partner's arm by the wrist with your nearside hand. Scoop your outside hand under the shoulder. Lean back slightly to stretch out the shoulder, then lift it and push it in over the ribs, then up toward the neck. Release and stretch back to begin again. Repeat three or four times.

11

Step 12

Place your partner's hand on the back. Ask your partner to "let go" both elbow and shoulder. Cup the outer shoulder with one hand and place the index finger of the other firmly alongside the shoulder blade border. Lift with the outer hand; lean in with the other, inserting the fingers under the blade for a moment. Release and repeat several times.

12

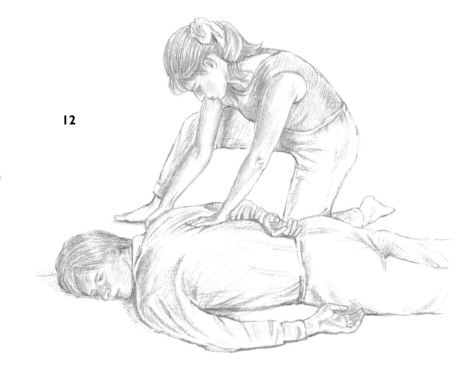

Step 13

Turn to face your partner. Palm down the Bladder Meridians on one side of the spine (see step 7 on page 97), using your other hand as support on the back. Repeat on the Bladder Meridian on the other side of the spine.

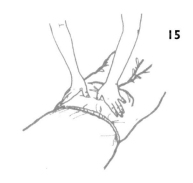

Step 14

If your partner has a very tense or muscular back, try using elbow pressure instead of palming. Position your elbows, relax your forearms, and gradually bring your weight forward to create perpendicular pressure. Ease back to shift your elbows, moving one a little ahead of the other as you follow the Meridian down the back. You can work both sides of the spine without changing position. Relax and take your time.

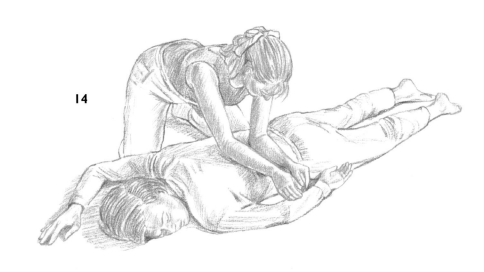

Step 15

Use both thumbs to apply pressure to the sacral points. They lie in two rows, one each side of the sacrum, in line with the main inner pathway of the Bladder Channel, and the other even closer to the midline.

BACK

Step 16

The buttock (gluteal) muscles are the largest in the body and they hold a lot of tension. Facing your partner, support yourself with one hand on the small of the back. With the flattened elbow of your other arm, lean into the buttock on the near side where you can let your weight sink comfortably. Then shift your weight forward into the other buttock, feeling your way into those spots that easily take your weight.

16

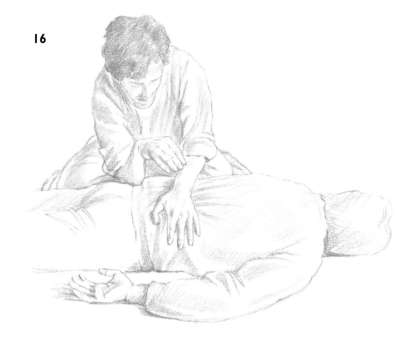

Step 17

Still leaning gently on your partner for support, step one foot over the thighs. Interlace your fingers and lean into each side of the sacrum. Reinforce the action by bringing your body forward. You may find it more comfortable to support one elbow with your leg, as shown.

17

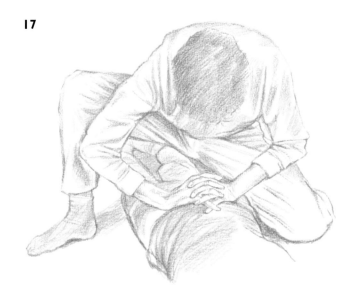

LEGS AND FEET

Check that your partner's ankles are relaxed so the feet contact the floor when you lean on the legs. If not, provide support with a small cushion or rolled towel.

Caution: *Do not massage B60 (on the outside of the ankle, see page 245) on anyone who is pregnant.*

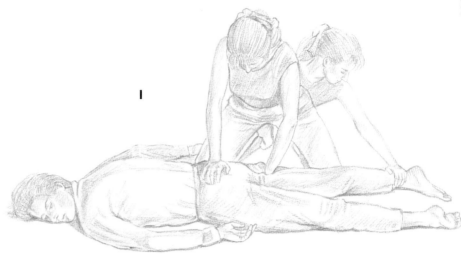

Step 1
Facing your partner, lean with your palm or heel of your hand over the midline of the thigh nearest to you, with your fingers pointing outward. Rest your other hand on the sacral region. Beginning under the buttocks, palm down the Bladder Meridian on the leg (see page 241). Before you reach the knee, turn your hand so your fingers are pointing away from you and continue palming. Work gently over the knee, and continue down the lower leg to the heel. Keep a wide base and avoid over-reaching.

Starting at the buttocks again, palm down the Kidney Meridian (see page 241) in the same way.

Step 2
Thumb the Bladder Meridian from the same position. Halfway down the calf the Bladder Meridian deviates outward slightly to run in the groove between the Achilles tendon and the ankle. Stop here on the outside of the foot.

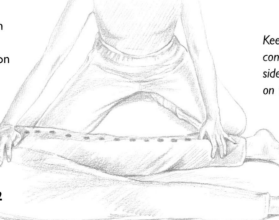

Keeping your supporting hand in contact, move round to the other side and repeat steps 1 and 2 on the other leg.

LEGS AND FEET

Work through steps 3 to 6 of this part of the sequence on one leg, then repeat on the other.

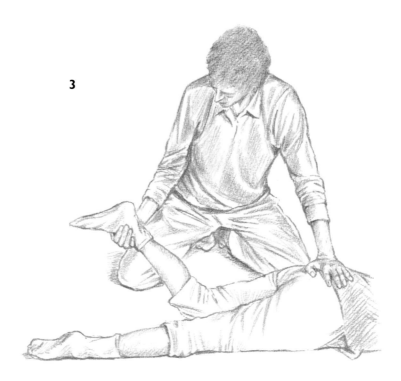

3

Step 3

With your support hand still resting on the sacrum, reach under your partner's ankle and lift the lower leg, stretching the knee and thigh.

Step 4

Fold the foot over toward the centre of the buttock. Lean gently but firmly, then slide your hand toward the toes to stretch the foot. Pause for a moment, then carry the foot back out to release the knee joint.

4

Step 5

Fold the leg across to the opposite buttock and stretch, following the movement with your body.

5

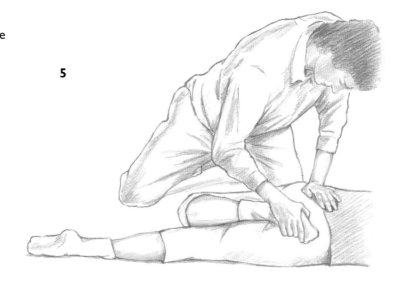

Step 6

Release the leg and carry it round in a circular movement, bringing the foot toward you and along the nearside of your partner's buttock. Then place the foot on the floor, toes pointing slightly inward.

6

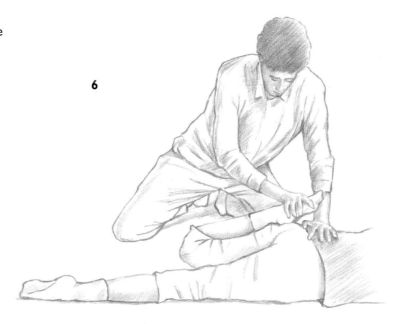

Move to the other side and repeat steps 3 to 6 on the other leg.

105

LEGS AND FEET

Step 7

Stand with the balls of your feet by your partner's toes. Keeping part of each foot in touch with the ground at all times, transfer your weight gradually on to your partner's feet. Shift from foot to foot to find comfortable positions.

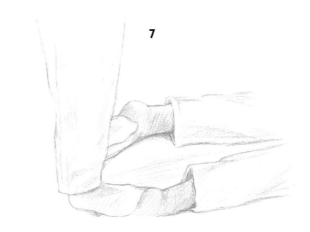

7

Step 8

Clasp under your partner's ankle with one hand as shown, keeping your hand on the floor for support. Then knead the whole underside of your partner's foot with the folded finger knuckles of the other hand, using your weight to apply a firm pressure. Repeat on the other foot.

Caution: *Do not use this step on anyone who is pregnant.*

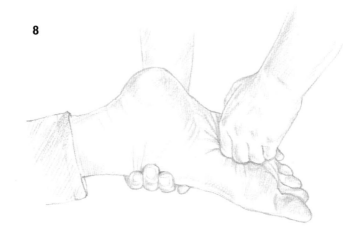

8

Now ask your partner to roll over on to her back for shiatsu on the front of the body. Use pillows or folded towels to ensure she is comfortable.

ARMS AND HANDS

Work through steps 1 to 12 of this part of the sequence on one arm, then repeat on the other.

Step 1

Kneel at your partner's side, facing the head. Rest your hand on the Hara (belly), with your fingertips above, and the heel of your hand below the navel. Relax your arm, do not lean or press. Observe, feel the breathing, and just "be" with your partner for a moment before starting. Even as a beginner, you can contact your partner's Ki at a deep level.

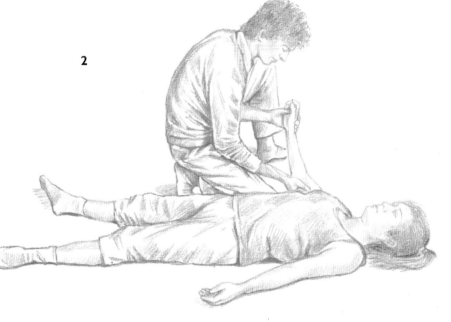

Step 2

Pick up your partner's arm by the hand or wrist, move your other hand from the Hara to the shoulder and, by leaning back slightly, stretch the arm out. Now move your near hand from the shoulder to the elbow and, carrying the arm, bend and rotate the forearm. If you feel your partner trying to help you by moving or holding the arm, gently encourage her to "let go".

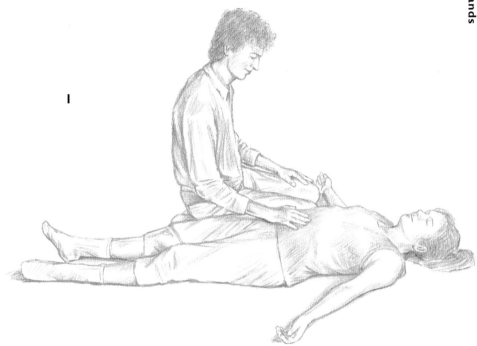

ARMS AND HANDS

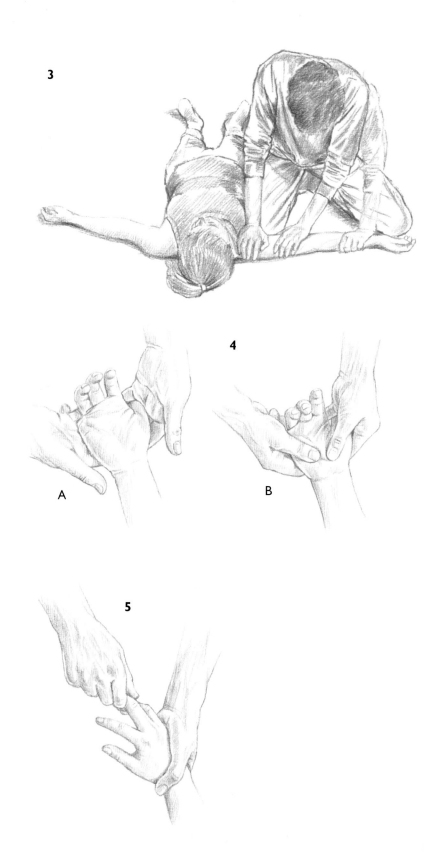

Step 3

Place your partner's arm on the floor at right angles to the body, with the palm and inner surface of the arm facing upward. Then, squatting, or kneeling up on your toes and keeping a wide base, lean with your support hand on to the front of the shoulder. Palm down the arm with the other hand, moving down inch by inch. Keep both hands relaxed, hugging the shape of the limb.

Step 4

Hold your partner's hand in both of yours, palm up and with the fingers toward you. Tuck your little fingers under the middle three fingers (A) supporting the hand with your other fingers. Then give thumb pressure systematically over the whole palm (B). You can rest the backs of your hands on your knees while you work.

Step 5

All the main Meridians end or begin on the fingers or toes. To stimulate the Meridian endings, squeeze the sides of the finger firmly between your thumb and the knuckle of your index finger. Work along each finger and thumb in stages, from knuckle to fingertip.

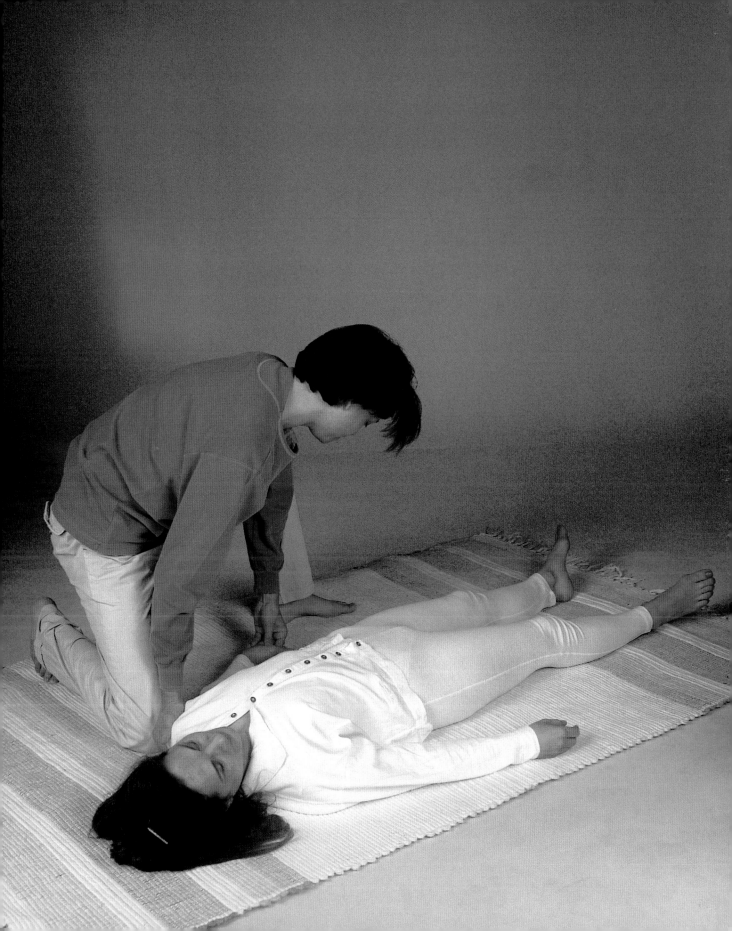

ARMS AND HANDS

Step 6
Pick up your partner's arm with your outside hand and with your other hand clasp the top of the shoulder. Lift the arm over your partner's head, then bring it round and down, out to the side, gently pulling on the wrist and shoulder to loosen the joints. Repeat a few times before placing the arm on the floor at 45 degrees to your partner's side.

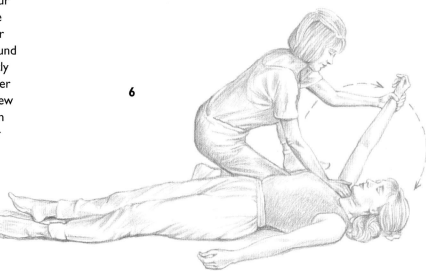

Step 7
In order to lean comfortably and contact the Ki of the Lung Meridian, move to the outside of the arm, facing in, with your partner's palm facing upward. Support your partner's shoulder with your nearside hand. Now lean into the hollow area at the front of the shoulder, corresponding to point Lu1 (see page 244) and place your other hand anywhere along the arm. Pause and relax for a few moments, knees spread wide.

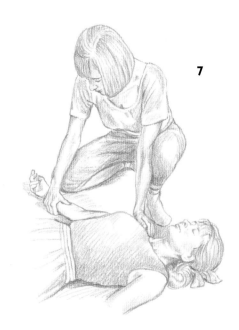

Step 8

Keep your nearside hand on the shoulder and with your other hand locate the biceps muscle. Lean your weight through the line of your extended thumb and the heel of your palm into the space between the muscle and the humerus bone. Ease up, slide your hand along two finger widths, then relax and repeat the pressure. Continue in this way on the near side of the arm, palming down the Lung Meridian to the wrist on the thumb side. Finish by gently squeezing along the sides of the thumb.

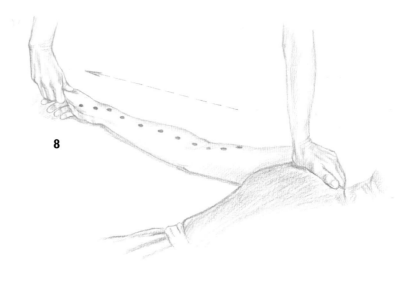

8

Step 9

Now, with your fingers supporting the arm, use your extended thumb to explore the groove between the biceps muscle and the bone. Slide your thumb along between these points, always keeping contact. Work into Lu5 on the outside of the biceps tendon at the elbow. Continue thumbing down the Lung Meridian to Lu9 at the base of the thumb.

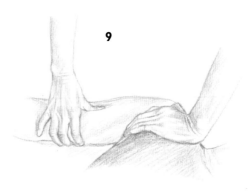

9

ARMS AND HANDS

Step 10

Thumb along the inside edge of your partner's thumb, including the point Lu10, found in the "belly" of the muscle at the base of the thumb. This is a sedating point for sore throats.

Step 11

Rotate your partner's hand slightly inward to bring the edge of the forearm uppermost. Lean on the outer part of your partner's shoulder with your support hand. Then gently grasp the upper arm with the other hand, and feel for the LI Meridian along the humerus bone (see step 12). Palm down this Meridian, moving your hand down in stages past the elbow, leaning and gently grasping, then along the bony edge of the forearm.

Step 12

Starting at the upper arm, work along the LI Meridian again with your flattened thumb. You may wish to use your thumb at a more penetrating angle to work the upper arm. Work down to LI11, at the outside end of the elbow crease when the arm is folded. Below the elbow use the "dragon's mouth" technique (see step 8 on page 97) to work down in stages from the elbow to the wrist.

Keeping one hand in contact, move to your partner's other side and repeat steps 1 to 12 on the other arm.

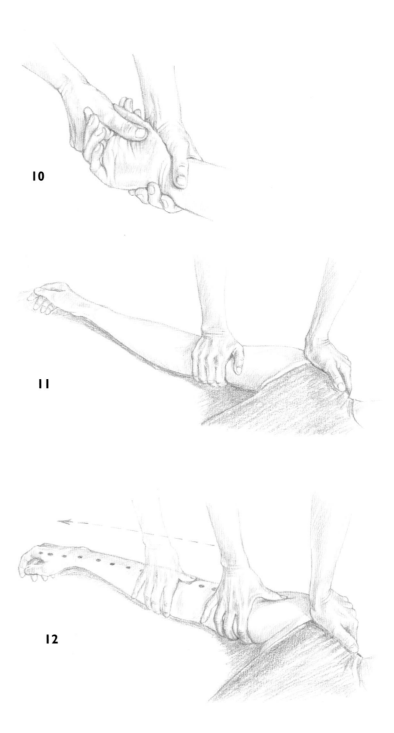

10

11

12

FACE

Step 1

Keeping a light contact at your partner's shoulder, move to a kneeling position behind your partner's head, with your knees spread wide either side of her ears. Lean both hands on your partner's shoulders and relax.

Rest the palms of your hands loosely over the temples and ears for a few moments. When you are ready, curl your fingertips to hold the occipital ridge at the base of the skull behind the ears. Roll the head gently a few times from side to side to loosen the neck. Then, resting the edges of your hands on the floor, move your fingers round under the head and curl the tips into the hollows beneath the occipital bone. Lean back from your Hara to open and stretch the neck, raising your partner's head slightly.

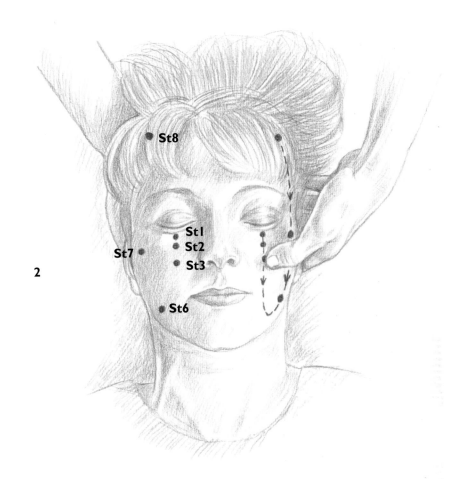

2

Step 2

Slide your palms underneath your partner's head, so it rests cupped in your hands. Pause here for a moment or two.

Roll your partner's head to the side, cradling and balancing it on your hand. The other hand is now free to work the Stomach Meridian along both its branches, with the thumb. Begin at St8, which is just inside the hairline at the corner of the forehead. The Meridian passes down the side of the head, about 2.5 cm (1 in) in front of the ear. Thumb along it, working into St7 under the cheek bone and St6 near the angle of the jaw in the middle of the powerful chewing muscle.

Then thumb along the other branch of this Meridian, which begins on the border of the eye socket at St1 and St2. St3 is under the cheek bone, level with the widest part of the nose.

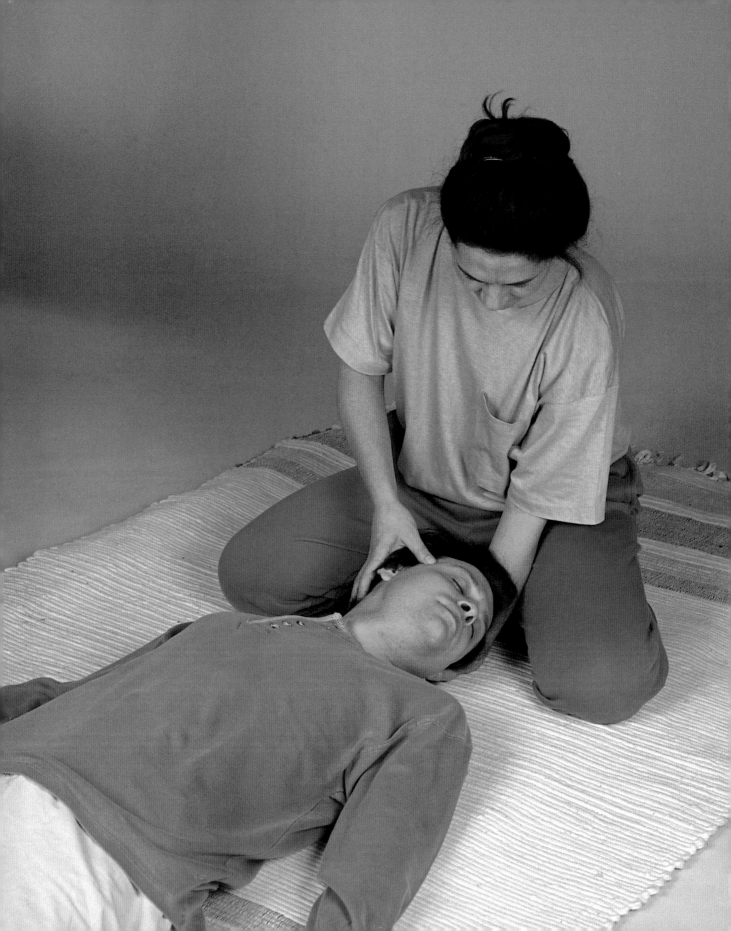

Step 3

LI 20, "Welcome Fragrance" is the last point of the Large Intestine Channel. Stimulating this point will help clear a sore stuffy nose or sinuses. Extend your index or little finger and lean at a slight angle upward and in toward the nose using the weight of your relaxed arm.

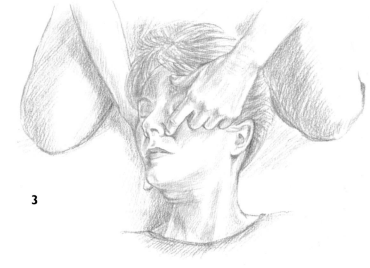

3

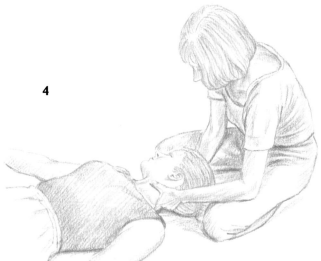

4

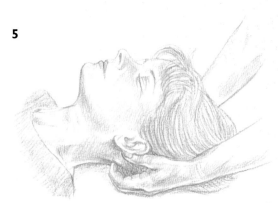

5

Step 4

Still cradling the head at a slight angle, work down the prominent muscle at the side of the neck. The LI Meridian runs along its top, and the Stomach Meridian a little to the front. Rest the ball of your thumb over the muscle, the fingers of your working hand supporting the back of your partner's neck. Try to feel as if your two hands are co-operating and connected. Alter the angle of your partner's head a little to promote relaxation, as you work down the muscle.

Step 5

Return your partner's head to centre. Slide your hands down under the head and overlap your fingers to encircle the underside of the neck below the skull, with your thumbs tucked against the jawbone. Lift up and back, gently arching the neck. Sink back from your hips to give a little stretch to the spine.

Replace the head on the floor, pulling back slightly on the occipital ridge under the skull. Finish this part of the sequence by leaning on to your partner's shoulders. Gently break contact after a few moments.

Repeat steps 2 to 5 on the other side of the face and neck.

LEGS

Work through steps 1 to 7 of this part of the sequence on one leg, then repeat on the other.

Step 1
Kneel facing your partner at hip level, your knees spread wide. Place one hand below the navel; the other, fingers pointing outward, on top of your partner's thigh. Palm down in stages to the knee, turning your fingers inward once you are below the level of the groin.

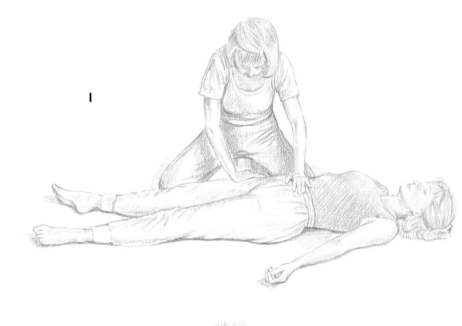

Step 2
Roll your partner's near leg inward and extend your own leg to rest the sole of your foot, heel on the ground, across the front of your partner's foot. This brings the Stomach Meridian uppermost. Then kneel up, bring your hips forward, and palm down the Meridian again, this time from the upper thigh to the lower leg.

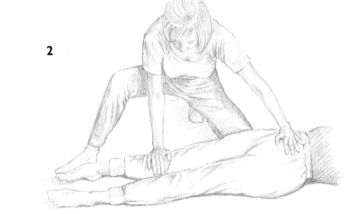

Step 3
From the same position thumb the Stomach Meridian down the leg. Slide your thumb down to St34, 5 cm (2 in) above the kneecap. Continue over the knee to St36, one hand's breadth below the kneecap, and down the leg, following the Stomach Meridian roughly one finger width outside the shinbone.

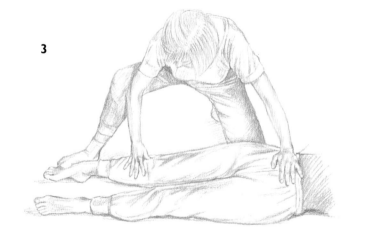

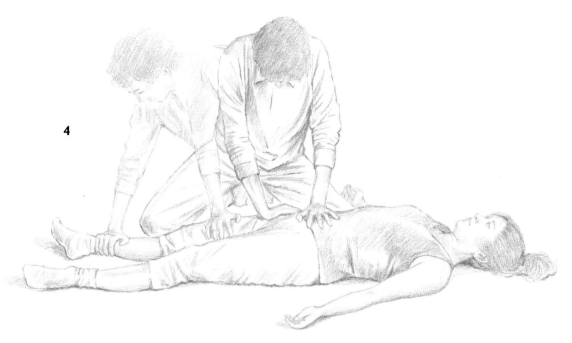

4

Step 4

Return your partner's leg to its natural position. With your support hand resting on the Hara, palm the near side of the leg past the knee to the ankle. On the lower leg, give more pressure to the outside of the shinbone through the heel of the hand, fingertips curled naturally over for support.

Bring your weight forward to palm down the inner aspect of the far leg. Keep the pressure of your support hand constant on the Hara as you rock back and forward to move and give pressure with your active hand. Palm down from thigh to ankle.

Step 5

Keeping your support hand on the Hara, reach around under the knee of the leg nearest you with the other. Lean forward to lift and bend the knee, with your partner's foot flat on the floor. Rest the bent leg against your side. Then bring your working hand out to push up on the front of the knee, lifting it up toward the abdomen. Rotate the hip inward and forward, around and back a few times, in a controlled way, using your body weight.

5

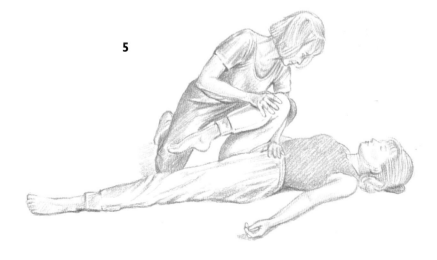

LEGS

Step 6

Lower your partner's leg against your body. Lift the ankle and slide the toes to the ankle of the other leg. Let your partner's knee fall gently outward. This brings the Spleen Meridian uppermost.

Caution: *Do not give shiatsu on the Spleen Meridian during pregnancy if miscarriages are likely. Do not use Sp6 (one hand width up from the inner ankle bone, see page 245) during any pregnancy.*

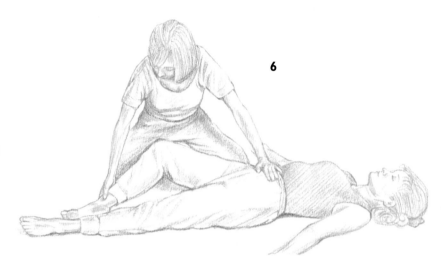

6

Step 7

Kneeling up and forward, support the knee on your thigh and lean on to your partner's inner thigh. Palm the Spleen Meridian past the inner edge of the kneecap to the ankle, starting with your fingers pointing outward and turning them inward as you work down the thigh.

7

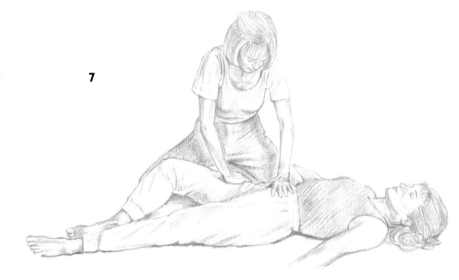

Keeping one hand in contact, move round to your partner's other side and repeat steps 1 to 7 on the other leg.

Step 8

Squat down close to your partner's feet, your knees wide outside your arms and your back as straight as possible. Reach down behind your partner's ankles to lift her heels a little off the floor. Pause and inhale.

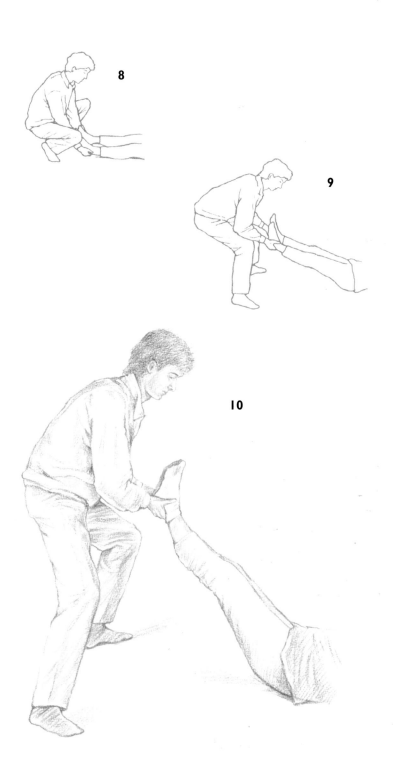

Step 9

In one smooth movement, keeping your back as straight as possible, exhale as you straighten your knees to lift your partner's legs to an angle of about 30 degrees. Step in a little to rest your arms on your thighs. Anchored by your partner's body weight, lean back to stretch the spine. Relax and breathe.

Step 10

When you are ready, begin to swing your partner's legs with small side-to-side rocking movements while still supporting your elbows. Then transfer your weight from foot to foot as you swing the legs and push the feet out, up, and away from you on each side. Do this only a few times before resting. Swinging the legs in a wide arc loosens the waist and lumbar region – a relief for tired, aching backs. Lower the legs carefully back to the floor. For your own sake keep your Hara low and your back straight.

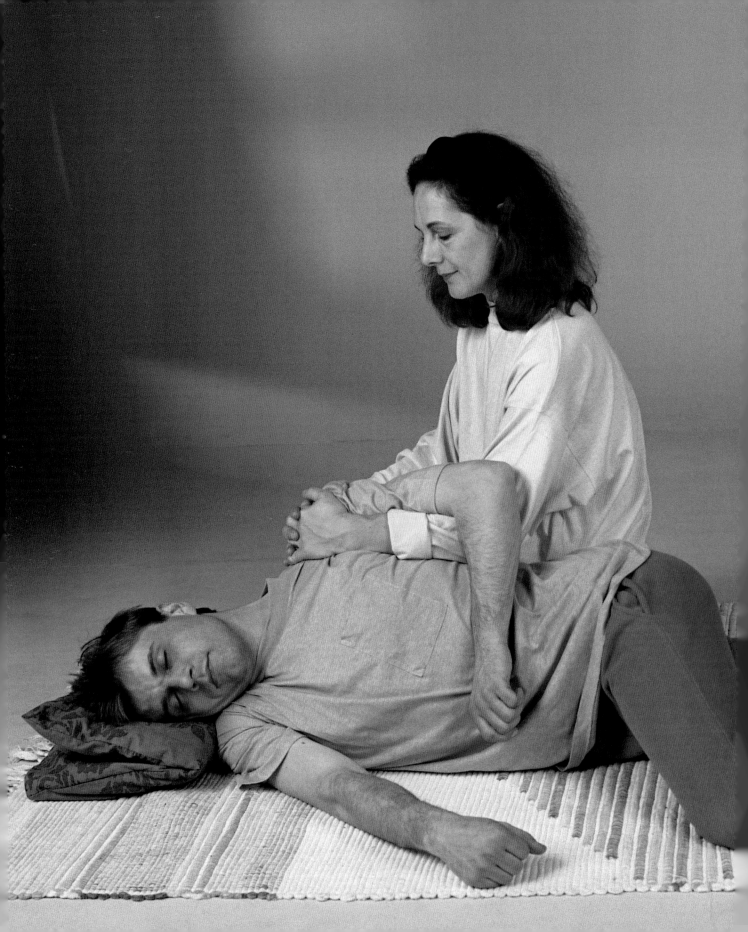

SIDE

Ask your partner to roll over on to one side. Use a pillow to support the head and find the most stable position by bringing the lower shoulder forward slightly to rest on the ground, and folding the top leg forward in front of the outstretched lower leg.

Work through steps 1 to 14 of this part of the sequence on one side, then repeat on the other.

Step 1

Kneel close by your partner's back, resting your nearside hand on the shoulder and placing your other between the shoulder blades, the area corresponding with the Heart and Pericardium. Pause here for a few moments.

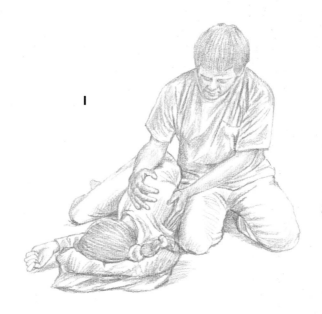

Step 2

Slide your arm into your partner's armpit to support the front of the shoulder. Clasp the shoulder with both hands and begin to move it slowly in circles. Follow and feel the limits of the motion and rotate the joint more widely, a few times in each direction.

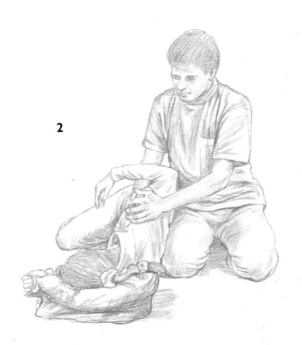

SIDE

Step 3

Palming the side of the head opens the Triple Warmer and Gall Bladder Meridians that cross it. Kneel up and step forward with your outer leg. Support your partner with the thigh of your near leg. Place your palms comfortably on your partner's head. Lean and palm gently around the side of the head.

3

Step 4

Tuck your near elbow against your partner's shoulder and place your hand behind the head. With your other hand, begin at T23, the small hollow near the outer end of the eyebrow, and follow the path of the Triple Warmer Meridian down to the front of the ear then back around the ear. Return to GB1, level with the outer corner of the eye, and thumb this Meridian down to the hollow in front of the ear, then around the ear and up to the forehead.

4

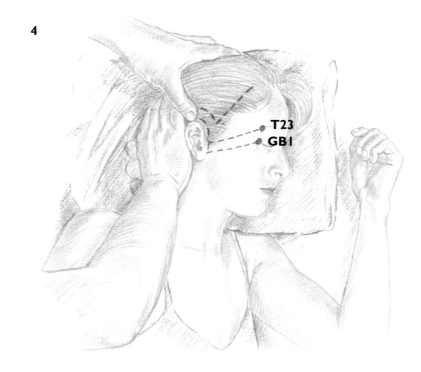

T23
GB1

Step 5

Sit back slightly and cup your support hand around the shoulder, then lean back a little to "open" the neck. With the fingers of your working hand give firm pressure to GB12 and GB20, under the base of the skull. Work down the side of the neck, at first just resting your thumb across the muscle using the relaxed weight of your arm. Then, working a little more firmly with extended thumb, give pressure behind the muscle along the Triple Warmer Meridian.

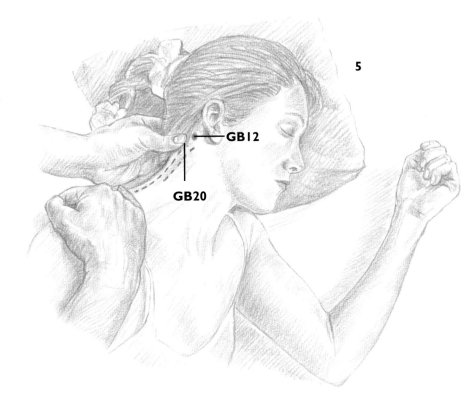

Step 6

Squat behind your partner's head. Rest your near hand over the head, curling your fingers under the base of the skull. With the thumb of the other hand work the Triple Warmer and Gall Bladder Meridians across the top of the shoulder (see page 241), inching along from the corner of the neck as far as the bony extremity.

Caution: *Do not massage GB21 (in the middle of the top of the shoulder, see page 242) on anyone who is pregnant.*

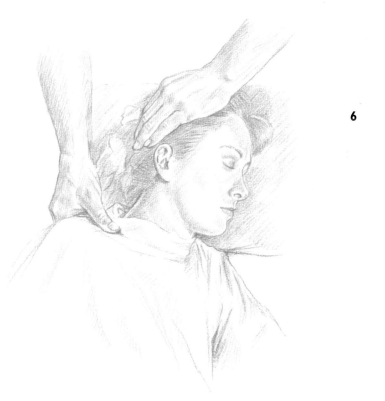

SIDE

Step 7

Kneeling alongside your partner's back, place your hands around the shoulder. Rock the joint loosely between your hands and feel for the inner border of the shoulder blade so that you can curl your fingers and hook them firmly under it. Supporting the front with equal pressure, lift up, out, and away from the spine by leaning back and opening your own body. This gives your partner a lovely releasing sensation. Repeat a couple of times.

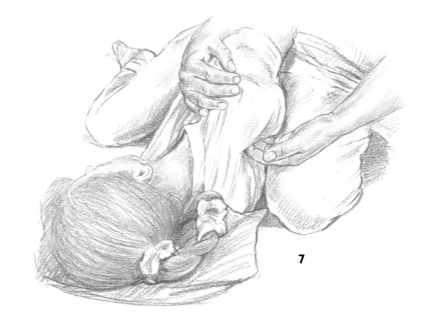

7

Step 8

Rest the arm along your partner's side, wrist over the hip. Kneel up behind, with your knees widely spaced, and steady your partner's shoulder with your supporting hand. Palm the outer arm from the shoulder muscle to the wrist. Then kneel back slightly to thumb the Triple Warmer Meridian in the upper arm. To follow the Meridian from the elbow, kneel up close and lean directly down, thumbing along the space between the two bones of the forearm to the hollow at the wrist where the tendons converge.

8

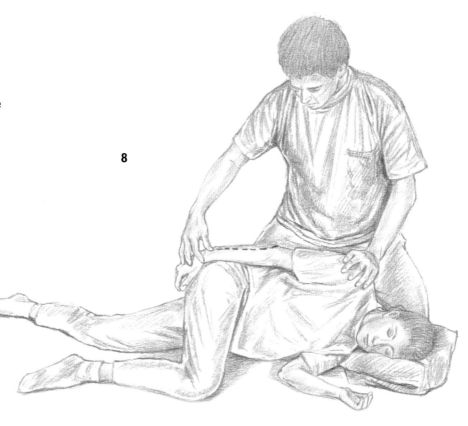

Step 9

Continue thumbing over the back of the hand, toward the space between the knuckles of the 4th and 5th fingers. Finish by squeezing the sides of the 4th finger.

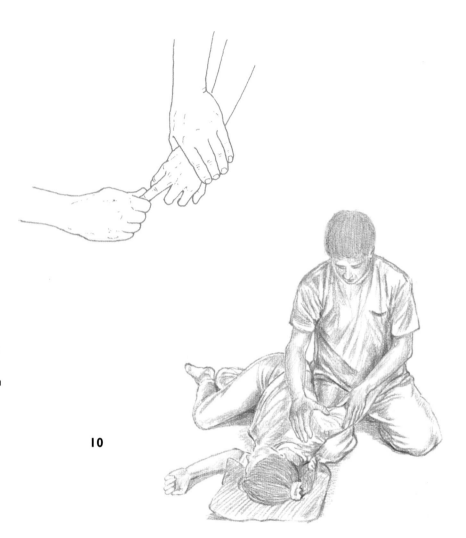

Step 10

Rotate your partner's shoulder backward, so her arm lies across your lap. First palm the Pericardium Channel (see page 241) with your thumb laid flat across the inner arm while your fingers support behind. Return to the top and thumb the Meridian at a more penetrating angle. Keep your shoulder relaxed.

10

Step 11

Lift and rotate the arm once or twice, then place it down in front of the body. Kneel up and place your hands so that the "V" between thumb and index finger is over the side of the ribcage. Lean in and use the dragon's mouth technique (see step 8 on page 97) to work down the Gall Bladder Meridian (see page 241), from the armpit to the waist. Keep both hands together and give your partner time to breathe with the movement.

11

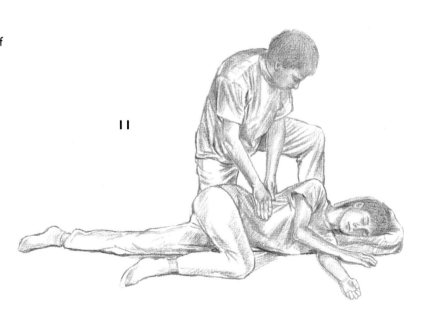

SIDE

Step 12

Step across your partner's legs as shown. Rest your supporting hand on GB30, on the outside of the buttock just above and behind the prominent hip bone. Palm down the middle of the outer leg from the hip to the ankle joint.

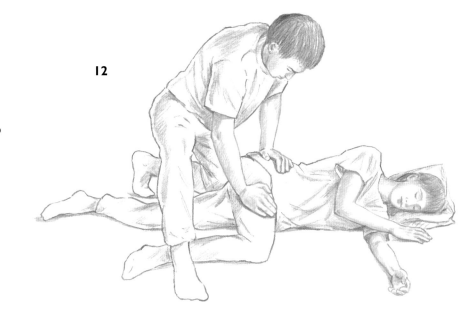

12

Step 13

Return to the buttock and thumb the Gall Bladder Meridian down to the knee. Below the knee, locate GB34 on the outside of the leg, 5 cm (2 in) below the kneecap, in the hollow immediately below and just in front of the head of the fibula. From here, work down toward the ankle, along the bony edge of the fibula. Cross in front of the ankle and thumb down to the space between the 4th and 5th toes.

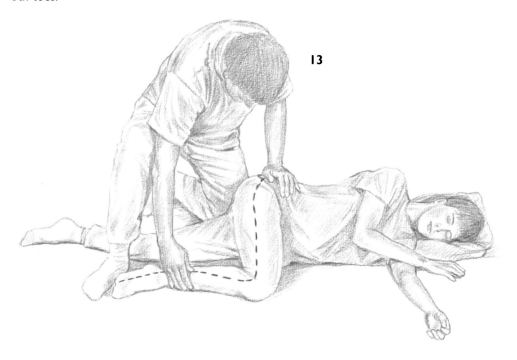

13

Step 14

Palm down the Liver Meridian on the inside leg, leaning into the relaxed tendon of the upper thigh, down past the knee and on to the calf, then close behind the bone on the lower leg to the ankle. Keep your support hand on the sacrum.

Then thumb along the Meridian, along the border of the tendon near the groin, then down the middle of the inner thigh to the knee. Work into Liv8, in the end of the knee crease.

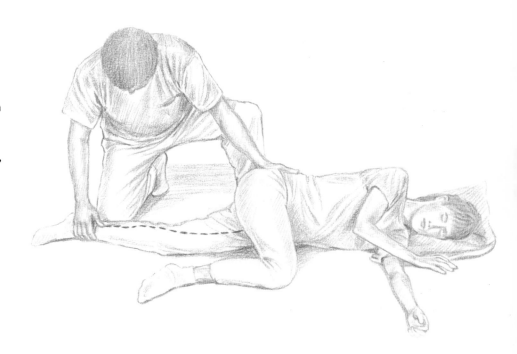

Ask your partner to roll on to her back and rest there briefly before rolling on to the other side. Repeat steps 1 to 14 on the other leg.

15

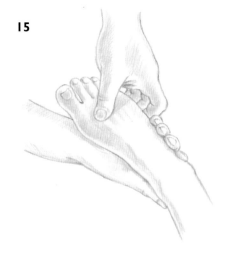

Step 15

Ask your partner to roll on to her back. Rotate each foot at the ankle joint, then grasp and stretch each one in turn, first away from the body, leaning back, then toward the head. Press Liv2 and Liv3 calmly and methodically on each foot. Hold the feet for a moment to finish.

Lay your hand gently on your partner's Hara and sit quietly for a few moments. Tell your partner gently that the work is done for now and leave her to rest quietly. You may wish to use the clearing visualization, or break the energy connection between you (see page 31).

CHAPTER 5

REIKI

The Reiki treatment described in this chapter works through the basic positions to treat the whole body. Reiki can also be used for distant healing; how to do this is described on pages 142–3.

When you receive a Reiki treatment, your emotions may be profoundly affected. Emotional "blocks" are often released and you come into closer contact with feelings you may have suppressed in the past – perhaps sadness or anger. It is important to accept these "negative" feelings. They are energies which can transform themselves into creative forces as soon as you "own" them and give them attention and expression. Before giving a Reiki treatment you should warn the receiver that they may have an emotional reaction. If this occurs, be ready to support your partner by listening, but try to avoid the temptation to "fix" their problems.

For the whole-body treatment, the receiver can sit on an upright chair or lie down – whichever is most comfortable. Reiki is usually given with the receiver clothed. Allow between 60 and 90 minutes for a full treatment; for elderly or sick people start with half an hour and increase the length of treatments gradually; for young children 10 to 20 minutes may be sufficient. Ideally start by giving four treatments on four consecutive days. This allows the body enough time to open itself on an energetic plane so it is able to free itself of its toxins more effectively. As it does so, chronic (long-term) disorders may again become acute. These self-healing reactions are a part of the healing process and mostly subside again within 24 hours. After the four treatment days, give further treatments once or twice a week, over several weeks. Remind the receiver to drink plenty after each treatment, to eliminate toxins.

Before starting the massage, prepare the room and centre yourself, following the guidelines on pages 28–30. Remind yourself that you are being used as a channel for healing energy and make the energy connection between you (see page 31). You may also wish to use the cleansing visualization (see page 30). At the beginning of the treatment, stroke the receiver's aura, holding your hands 15 cm (6 in) from the body, starting at the head and working down to the feet. This relaxes and prepares the receiver for treatment.

Caution: *See page 5 for a full list of cautions and contraindications for massage.*

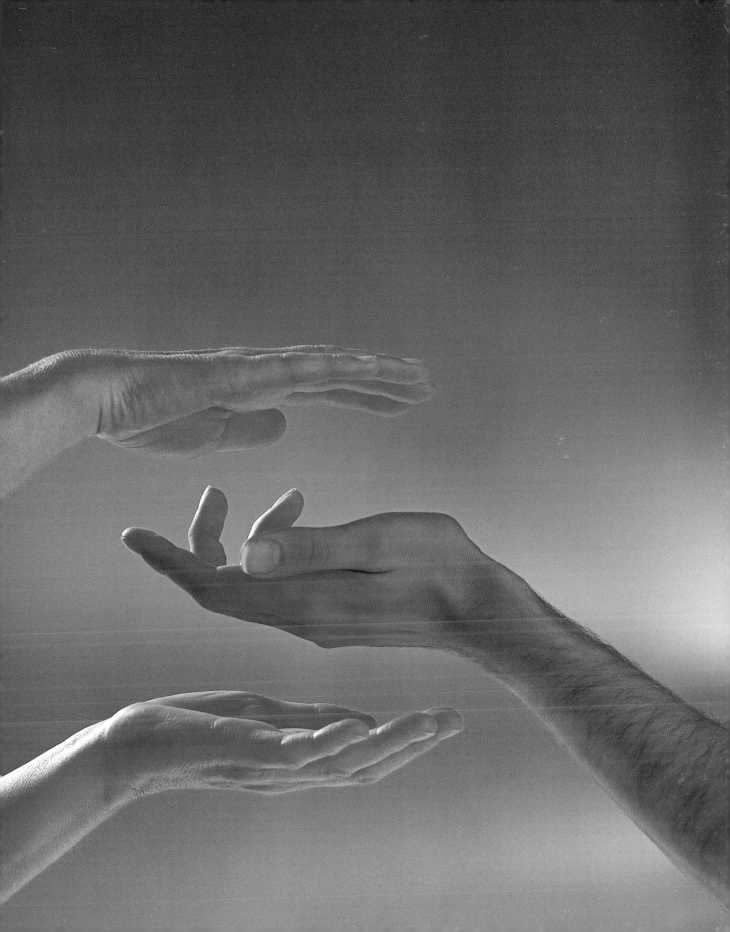

HEAD

*Hold your hands in each position for
3 to 5 minutes. Focus your intention by
visualizing a beam of energy, in the
form of a healing light, flowing down
from the universe, through you, and out
of your hands into the receiver.*

Step 1
Place your hands on your partner's
face, either side of the nose,
covering the forehead, eyes, and
cheeks. Relaxing the eyes relaxes
the whole body. If your partner
wishes, you can spread a tissue over
the forehead and out to the tip of
the nose, before placing your hands.

Step 2
Place your hands on the temples,
with the fingertips touching the
cheekbones, palms following the
shape of the head. This position is
good for treating the eye muscles
and nerves. It balances the right and
left sides of the brain, and the body.

Step 3
Place your hands over the ears. This
position is good for treating the
organs of balance and the pharynx.

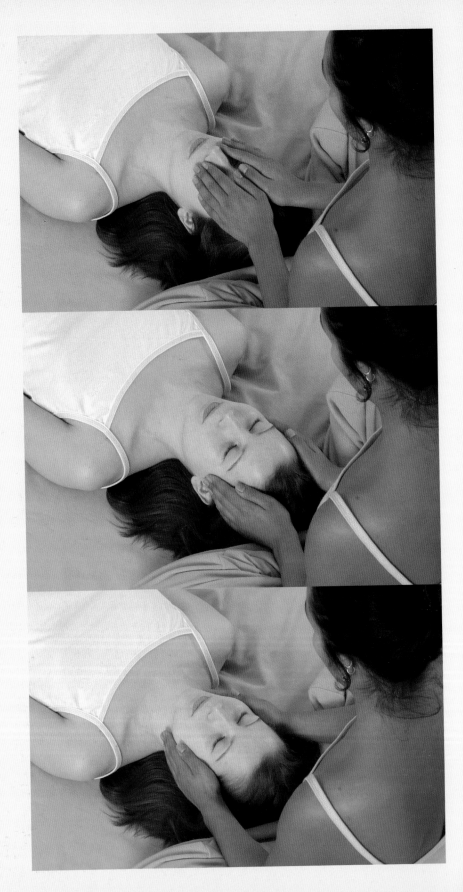

Step 4

Hold the back of the head with the fingertips over the base of the skull. This position is good for treating the back of the head, eyes, and nose and to calm and clarify thinking.

Step 5

Place your hands on the top of the chest, below the front part of the throat, without touching the throat directly. This position is good for treating the thyroid and parathyroid glands, larynx, vocal cords, and lymph nodes and to promote self-expression.

Step 6

Place both hands on the cap of the skull. This position is good for harmonizing the right and left sides of the brain and calming both mind and body.

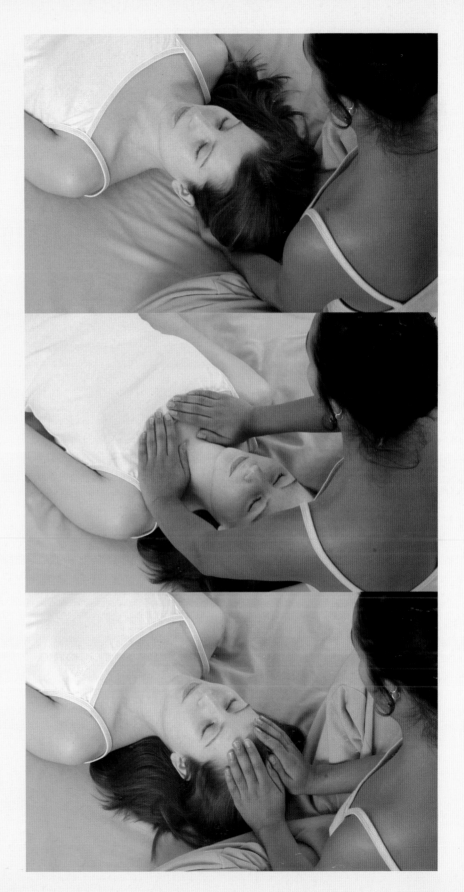

FRONT OF BODY

By treating the front of the body, you deepen the whole healing process. Emotional reactions are quite possible, though they are not inevitable. As you apply Reiki here you balance the organs and stimulate the Chakras on the front of the body (see page 251).

Step 1

Lay one hand across the upper chest below the collarbone, the other at right angles to the first on the breastbone in the middle of the chest, in a "T" shape. This position is good for treating the thymus gland, heart, and lungs. It is related to the heart (fourth) Chakra.

Step 2

Lay one hand on the lower ribs on your partner's right side, the other directly below it at waist level. This position is good for treating the liver and gallbladder, pancreas, duodenum, and parts of the stomach and large intestine. It also balances emotions such as anger and depression.

Then move your hands across the body to the same position on your partner's left side. This is good for treating the spleen, parts of the pancreas, large intestine, small intestine, and stomach, and helps to stabilize the immune system.

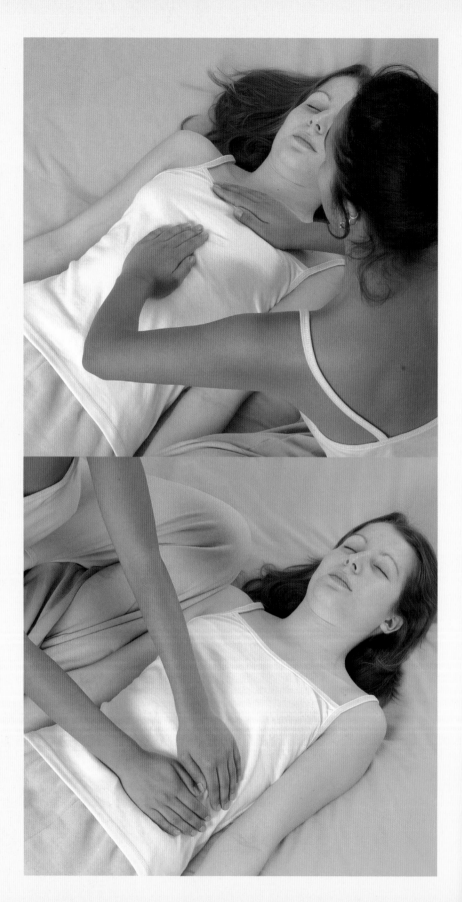

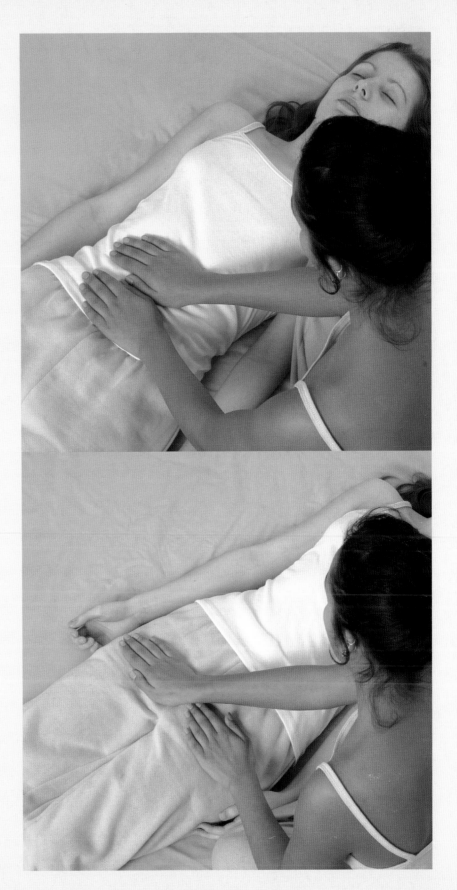

Step 3

Place one hand above, and the other below, the navel. This position is good for treating the solar plexus, stomach, digestive organs, lymphatic system, and intestines. Related to the sacral (second) and solar plexus (third) Chakras, it is also very good for restoring energy and vitality.

Step 4

For men, place your hands in the groin area, without touching the male organ. For women, lay both hands over the pubic bone. This position is good for treating the abdominal organs, intestines, bladder, and urethra. It is related to the root (first) Chakra.

FRONT OF BODY

Step 5

Lay your hands across the upper chest, fingers pointing outward. This position helps to harmonize the male and female sides.

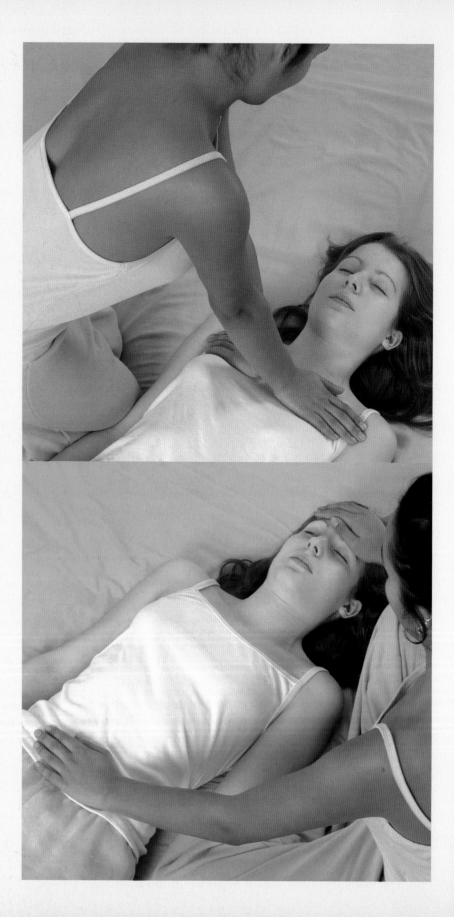

Step 6

Lay one hand on the forehead and the other on the belly (just below the navel). This position has a calming and centring effect. It promotes spiritual equilibrium and relaxes those suffering from stress.

Step 7

Place your hands on your partner's hips. This position is good for treating the hip joints, varicose veins, and leg pain.

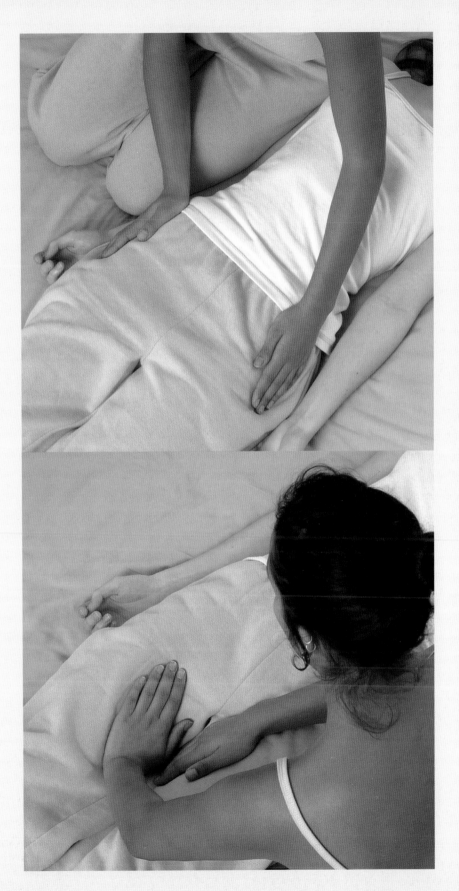

Step 8

Lay one hand flat on the inside of each thigh, with your fingertips pointing in opposite directions. This is a let-go position for deep-seated fears – emotions and tensions are released.

135

BACK OF BODY

Treating the back allows further letting go of tensions, thoughts, and feelings. Lying on the front of the body makes the receiver feel more protected, so healing and relaxation can take place at deeper levels.

Step 1

Place one hand on the nape of the neck and the other just below it at the top of the spine. This position treats pain in the bones, and heart, spine, nerve, and neck problems.

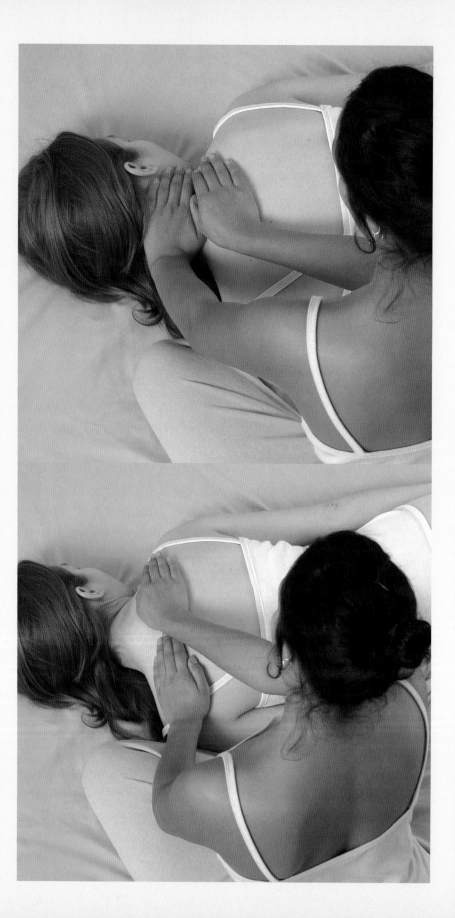

Step 2

Lay both hands on the shoulders, one hand to the left and the other to the right of the spine, fingers pointing in the same direction. This position eases tension in the shoulders and the nape of the neck.

Step 3

Move your hands down to the shoulder blades. This position is good for treating the shoulders, heart, lungs, and upper back. It promotes the capacity for love, confidence, and enjoyment.

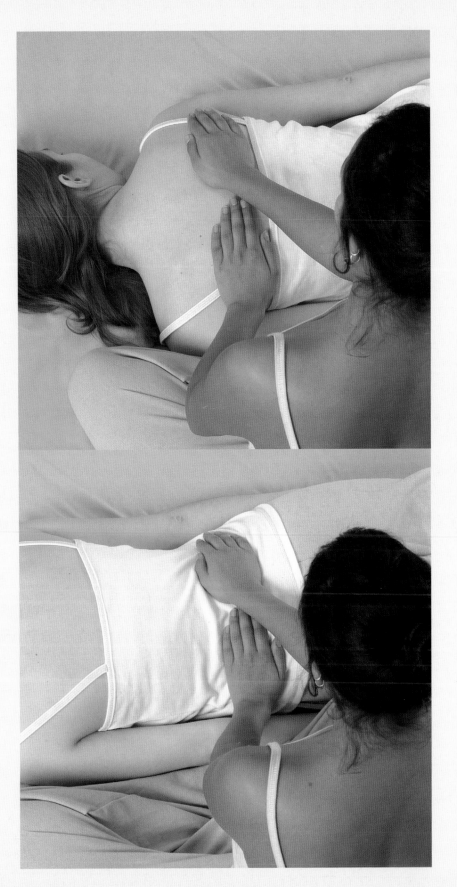

Step 4

Lay your hands on the lower ribs above the kidneys. This position helps in the treatment of the adrenal glands, kidneys, and nervous system. Then move your hands down to waist level. By releasing the middle back we let go of the past, of stress and pain.

BACK OF BODY

Step 5

Place your hands on the lower part of the back, at hip level. This position strengthens the lymph and nerves, and also supports creativity and sexuality.

Step 6

Lay your hands on the upper spine, one above the other, fingers pointing toward the head. Then move your hands down to the lower spine, still keeping one above the other. These positions treat back problems and disc wear.

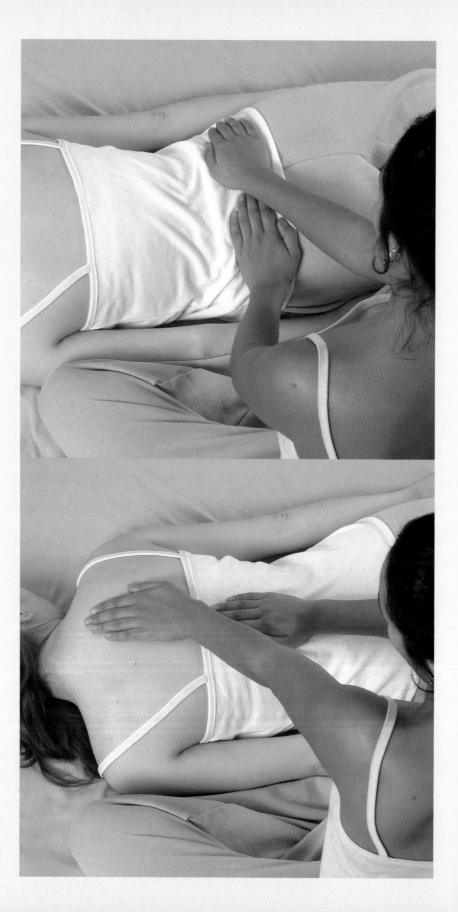

Step 7

Lay one hand across the sacrum, the other at right angles to the first, over the coccyx to form a "T". This position is good for treating the intestines, the urogenital system, and the sciatic nerve. It is related to the root (first) Chakra and helps to calm existential fears.

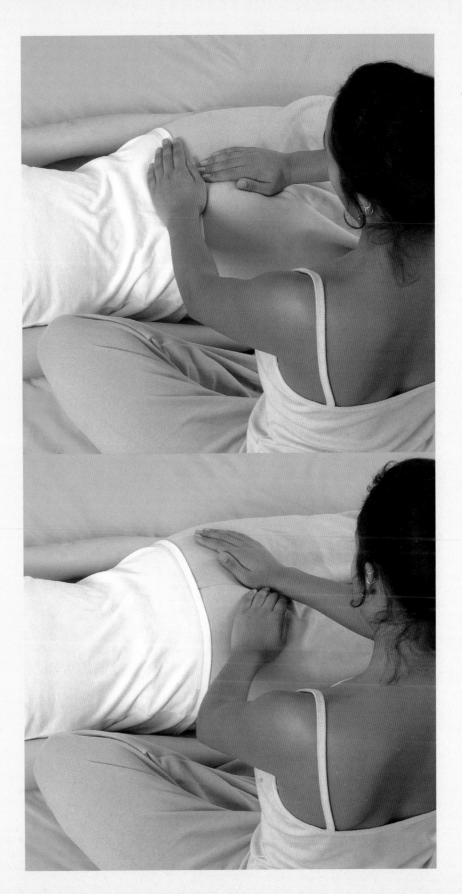

Step 8

Lay the fingertips of one hand directly on the coccyx (sometimes you will have to feel around a bit to find this bone). Lay your other hand next to the first to form a "V" shape. This treatment is the same as for step 7, but with the fingertips directly on the coccyx, the energy can more easily travel up the spine to energize and harmonize the nervous system, promoting confidence.

LEGS AND FEET

The legs and feet carry the whole weight of the body. Problems with the legs, knees, and feet can indicate a fear of moving forward in life. We also store emotions in the upper and lower leg areas. Reiki can release this energy and bring awareness to take the right steps in the right direction.

Step 1
Cover the hollows of the knees with your hands. This position is good for treating all parts of the knee joints, and fear, especially fear of dying.

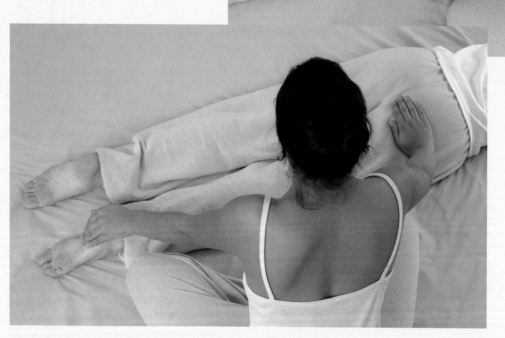

Step 2
Lay one hand on the buttock and the other on the heel on the same side. Then repeat on the other side. This position is good for treating sciatic pain.

Step 3

Place your hands on the soles of the feet, with your fingertips on the toes. This position is good for treating the foot reflex zones for all the organs, which are located over the whole sole (see pages 246–7). It fortifies the root (first) Chakra and grounds all the Chakras and regions of the body.

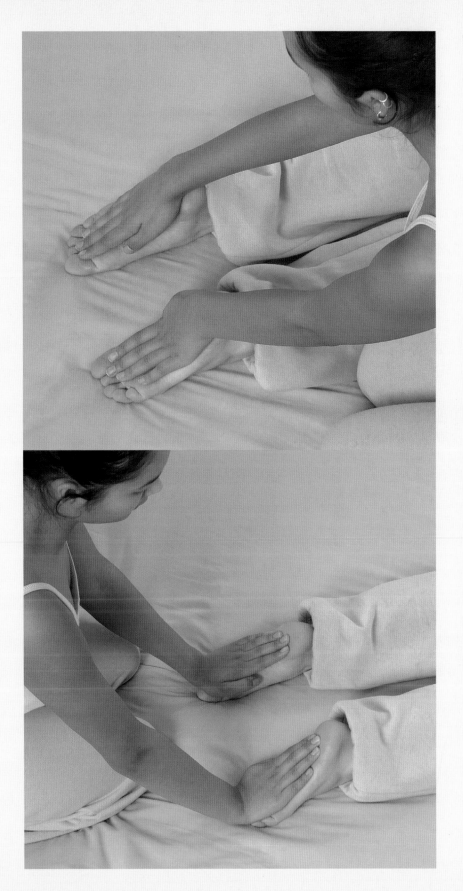

Step 4

Rest the heels of your hands on the toes and point your fingertips toward the heels. This position has the same effect as step 3. The receiver will sense a strengthening energy flow from feet to head.

End the treatment by smoothing your partner's aura three times, holding your palms about 15 cm (6 in) from the body. Break the energy connection between you (see page 31) and leave your partner to rest, covered with a blanket or towel.

DISTANT HEALING

This form of healing lets you send mental messages and healing forces over a distance. This is similar to the phenomenon of thought transference. How often have you thought about someone and then received a letter or phone call from him or her that very day? An incident like this may seem like mere coincidence, but it is proof that thoughts are transmitted and received on the mental level (telepathy).

You can give distant healing using visualization (see facing page) and transmit the healing energy to the receiver as if over a "bridge of light", over long distances. The healing power may be greatly amplified during distant healing, because the mental forces are very strong.

Ideally, you should agree the treatment time for a distant healing in advance and the receiver should sit or lie down, since it is better for him or her not to be doing anything. If you do not know your receiver personally, you can use a photograph to help visualize where you are focusing your attention. Allow 15 to 30 minutes for the distant healing session.

You can use distant healing whenever, for reasons of time or distance, you are unable to treat the receiver in person. Always ask the receiver at the start of the mental contact whether they want to receive healing from you. Reiki is a non-intrusive healing method. If people do not want to receive it, then you should respect their wishes. In general, the best advice is to wait until you are asked before you send Reiki.

Healing the planet
In times of general unrest, during disasters and wars, you can send Reiki to the whole Earth, or concentrate on a specific region.

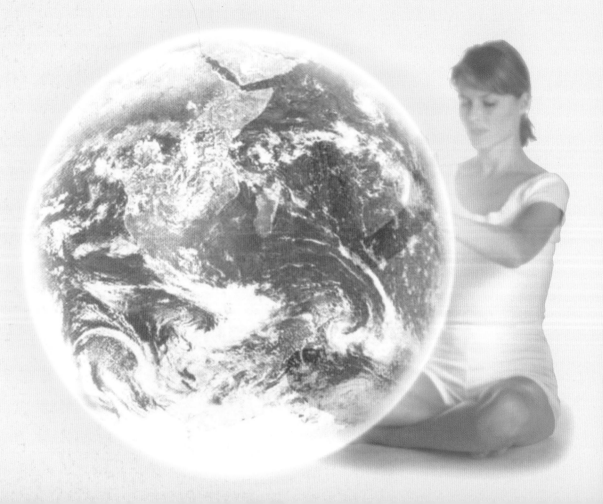

DISTANT HEALING VISUALIZATION

In this exercise you send Reiki or loving and healing thoughts across a distance.

Imagine that you are full of a golden light that charges your whole body and radiates from it. This light encases you like a protective shell.

Now "feel" or "see" the person to whom you wish to send healing. Once the person "appears", he or she is also included in the light.

Now send the light energy from the palms of your hands to the person to be treated. Direct the palms of your hands toward your visualization of the person. Imagine two laser-like beams of light flowing as healing energy from your palms into the body of the receiver. You can also imagine sending loving and healing thoughts to that person.

Continue for about 30 minutes. As you become more practised and sensitive to the flow of energy, you will be able to feel it drop away when the session is complete.

At the end of the exercise imagine the golden light that encompassed both of you slowly dispersing.

Caution

Distant healing must never be sent to anyone undergoing an operation, since it can undermine the effects of the anaesthetic. However, it can be used safely both in preparation for the operation and to assist natural healing processes afterward.

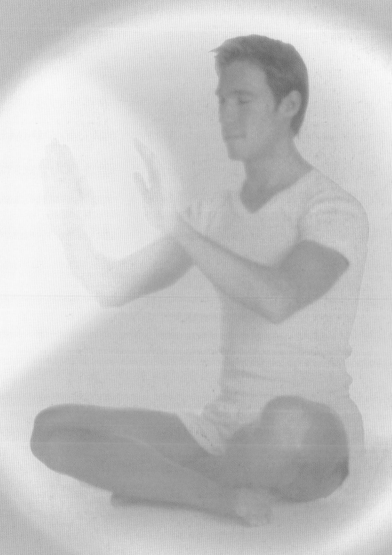

CHAPTER 6

INTUITIVE MASSAGE

An intuitive massage creates feelings of wellbeing, trust, and joy. It can also release a great deal of energy hitherto wasted in tension, and by transforming chronic habits of acting and reacting, effect profound changes on both posture and facial expression. On a spiritual level, it is not uncommon during an "intuitive" massage for both giver and receiver to attain a state of heightened awareness, of "presence in the moment", akin to the experience of meditation.

In intuitive massage the attitude of both giver and receiver, and the communication between them, are of paramount importance. The receiver's role is to be relaxed but alert, concentrating on the giver's touch. As giver you should remain centred and give your partner your full attention, for the healing energy transmitted through your hands will be weakened or deflected by an absent mind. When you are centred, you are guided by your intuition and will more readily sense where the sources of tension or energy imbalance lie. If your thoughts start to drift, simply bring them gently back and quieten your mind by concentrating on your breathing. Working with your eyes closed for brief periods may help you to stay in touch and keep your attention focused in your hands.

Clearly, it is not in the spirit of intuitive massage to provide step-by-step instructions. Page 146 describes the key elements of a basic holistic massage sequence. Following your intuition when treating each area of the body in turn will make sure that no areas are overlooked. The two meditations on pages 148–9, which can be used before giving any type of massage, will help to strengthen your connectedness to your intuition and Higher Self. Your intuition can tell you where to place your hand on the receiver's body. Simply ask, "Where are my hands needed right now?" and trust the first answer that comes into your mind. The Reiki sequence on pages 150–51 suggests a framework for a complete intuitive treatment.

The shiatsu techniques described on pages 152–3, for deepening the energy connection between giver and receiver, and working from the Hara (belly), can also be used with any type of massage to increase awareness, intuition, power of healing, and trust.

Before you begin, prepare the room and yourself, and any oils you wish to use, following the guidelines on pages 28–30.

Caution: *See page 5 for a full list of cautions and contraindications for massage.*

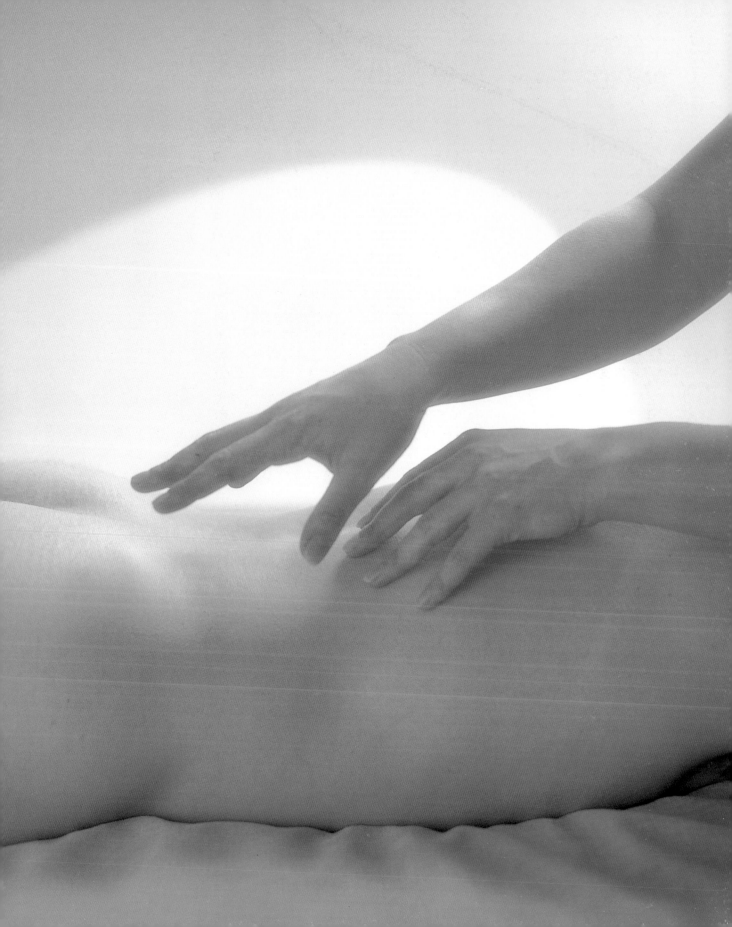

INTUITIVE HOLISTIC MASSAGE

This basic massage sequence checklist will help to ensure that you massage each part of the body in turn. Remember to oil the part of the body you are working on. Then begin with light, broad strokes, moving on to deeper ones, and finishing with lighter ones again.

Back
First work broadly over the whole area, then concentrate on the smaller portions in turn: the shoulder blades and upper back; the lower back, buttocks, and sides of the torso; and finally, the spine itself.

Back of legs
Work up one leg, then knead your way down it. End by massaging the foot. Repeat on the other leg.

Shoulders, neck, and scalp
With your partner lying on her back, begin with the shoulders, working on both front and back at once. Next, turn the head to one side to work on each shoulder separately. Then massage all over the scalp.

Face
Start at the forehead and travel down to the chin, working outward from the centre to the sides. Give the eyes, nose, jaw muscles, and ears special attention.

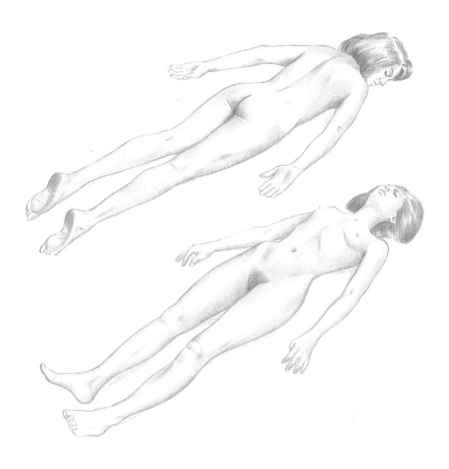

Arms and hands
Work up the arm and then knead down it again. End by massaging the wrist and hand. Repeat on the other arm.

Front of torso
Begin by focusing on the ribcage and sides of the torso. Then move down, circling around the abdomen. Finish by working up from the belly with long, sweeping strokes.

Front of legs
Work up the front of the leg, circling the kneecap on the way, then knead down the leg again. End by massaging the foot. Repeat on the other leg.

Connecting
Finally link all the parts of the body, either by using long "connecting" strokes or by resting your hands briefly on two separate parts of the body (see page 66).

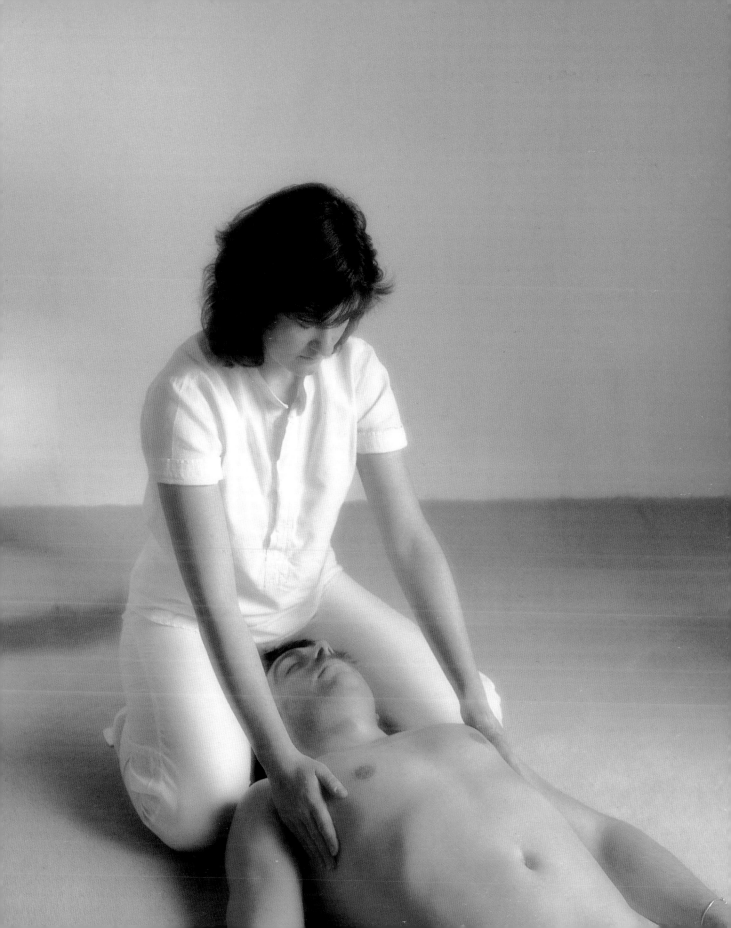

MEDITATION TO STILL YOUR MIND

Using one of the meditations on these two pages before you give intuitive massage will help you get into the rhythm more easily.

Step 1

You can either sit in a chair or lie down. Breathe in deeply through the nose and out through the mouth, making a light sigh on each exhalation. Let go of any tension to try to gain a sense of relaxation throughout your whole body.

Step 2

Place the palms of your hands gently over your eyes. After about 3 minutes in this position, bring your awareness down into your feet. Now start watching, with your eyes still closed, the energy emanating from this area. If you sense any tension in them, try to release it. Continue to do this until you feel completely relaxed and at ease.

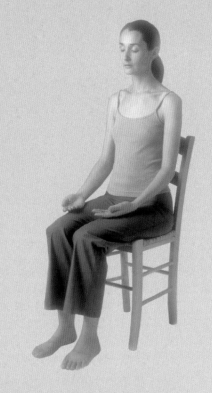

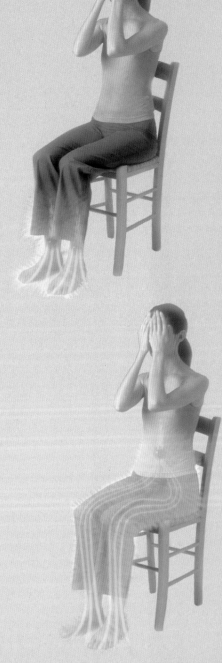

Step 3

Now move your awareness to your legs and try to tap into any tension there. Again, if you do find tension, aim to relax the affected areas.

Then focus awareness on all the other parts of your body in turn. Work mindfully through the groin area, stomach, buttocks, hips, shoulders, arms and all the organs. Then bring your attention to your hands, which are closely connected with your state of mind. If your left hand is tense, for example, the right side of your brain tends to be tense and vice versa.

Finally, relax your whole face, head and neck. Feel any tension in your mind and visualize it just melting away, bit by bit. Often this process will cause the tension and anxiety to simply pass on by.

MEDITATION TO DEVELOP SENSITIVITY

This exercise develops your ability to tap into your own energy field and heightens your awareness of your aura (electromagnetic field).

Step 1
Sit somewhere comfortable, with your back straight. Close your eyes for a few moments and consciously try to relax your shoulders on each of three out-breaths. As you do this, let go of any thoughts and tensions that you are aware of in the body.

Step 2
Now hold your hands in front of you, with your palms facing each other, about 30 cm (12 in) apart. Breathe in and out deeply through your belly. Watch from inside, with your eyes closed, how the energy builds up between your hands. Do this for 2–5 minutes.

Step 3
Gradually move your hands toward each other, becoming aware of the energy field between your hands. You are likely to feel resistance the more you practise this.

Step 4
Move your hands closer together, then further away from each other and back in. Notice how this feels. You might experience a tingling or tickling sensation, like static electricity, or you might feel a kind of pressure building up between your hands. Each person senses their energy in a unique way.

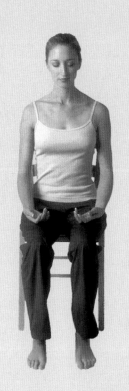
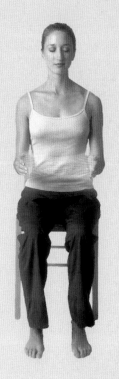
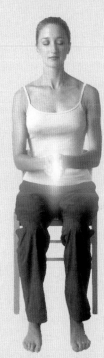
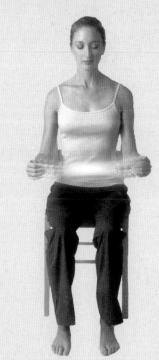

INTUITIVE REIKI

This "expanded" form of Reiki treatment allows you, as the giver, to connect with your intuition. You allow your hands to move wherever they are drawn. This often indicates an area where there is tension, a lack of energy, an imbalance, or a pain that needs to be released.

The receiver should lie down, either on a blanket on the floor or on a treatment table. Have another blanket nearby. Allow 30–40 minutes for the treatment.

Step 1

Sit behind your partner's head. Connect with your centre (see the centring meditation on page 30) and empty yourself of thoughts, tensions, and feelings. With each of your out-breaths, let go a little more and breathe out any tension.

Step 2

Tune in from your heart. With both hands, gently touch the receiver's head above the ears. Close your eyes. Now be receptive and open yourself to receive any information or message from the receiver. A "message" is where you feel a need for the receiver's body to be touched in a certain place. Messages can include visual pictures, sounds, or words that tell you something about the emotional wellbeing of the receiver.

Follow your intuition and place your hands. Wait until you feel like continuing.

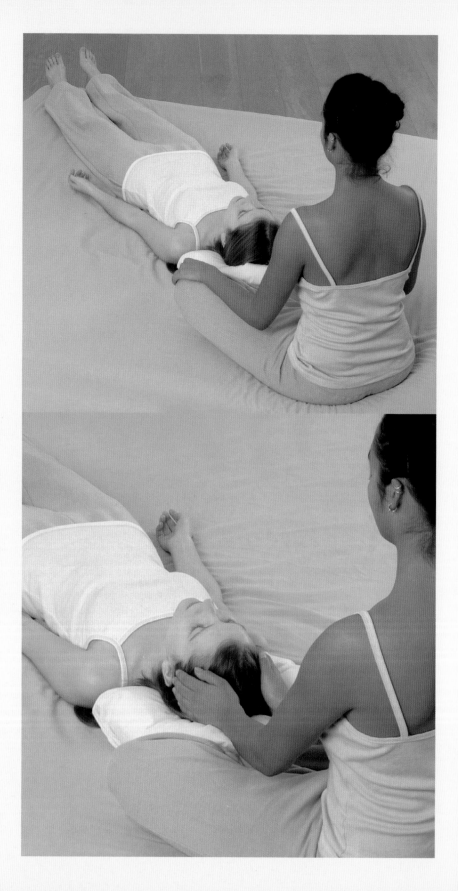

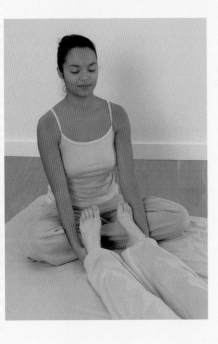

Step 3

Now go to the receiver's feet. Hold the heels in each hand. Close your eyes. Take a deep breath or two and connect with your own centre. Relax and open yourself to accept any information from the receiver's body. Get a clear picture of where the person wants to be touched. You may notice tingling in your hands.

Follow your intuition and place your hands. Wait until you feel like continuing.

Step 4

Sit on one side of the body at the level of the receiver's waist. With eyes closed, tune in and connect with the receiver. Hold one of her hands and wait for the contact between you to build. Place your hands where your intuition tells you. Wait until the impulse to move on comes.

Step 5

Now place your hands on the body, wherever you feel drawn. Use your inspiration and intuition to know where the body needs healing and continue with Reiki treatment.

At the end of the treatment hold the receiver's feet for a short time. Cover her with a blanket, and allow time for returning to normal consciousness.

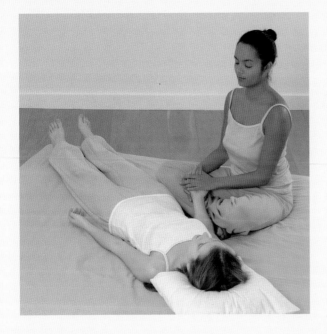

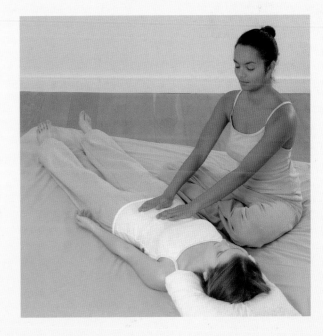

DEVELOPING A DEEP ENERGY CONNECTION

The techniques on these two pages will strengthen and deepen your shiatsu. They can also have a powerful effect when incorporated in other types of massage.

Two hands connection

Shiatsu encompasses support, which has a Yin quality, and the Yang, dynamic aspect of movement. The giver's two hands harmonize these Yin and Yang aspects. With practice you will begin to feel their unifying power in the receiver's response.

One hand fulfils the supportive function for both giver and receiver. Remaining stationary, it contacts the receiver's "centres of energy" and is sometimes called the "listening" or "parent" hand. The more active hand, sometimes known as the "child", follows the Ki in its movement round the body, innocently exploring the receiver's condition. Either hand can play the supporting role, as long as the parent and child are "in touch" with each other.

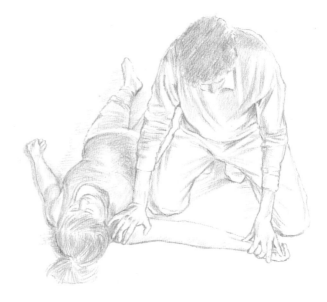

Continuity

A feeling of flow and continuity is essential to enhance your partner's experience of shiatsu. Continuity depends on your movements and the focus of your mind.

Concentrate on using your hands fluently as you work around your partner's body. Follow the Ki in its Channels by sliding your active hand along without breaking contact, to feel its condition. Move or pause as necessary, always maintaining contact with your support hand.

Focus your attention on your partner's breathing, and work from your Hara (see facing page). When your body and mind act in concert, your partner will be unaware of your technique but will experience the shiatsu as being deeply nourishing. Good continuity depends on your ability to work from the Hara.

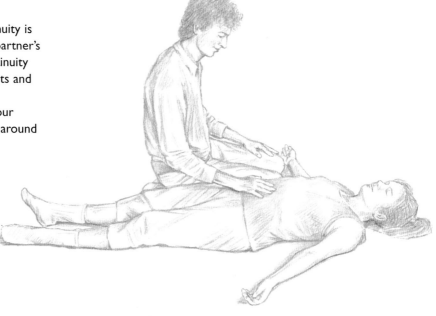

WORKING FROM THE HARA

Your Hara is in your belly, or abdomen. It is not only your physical centre of gravity but the seat of your constitutional energy or life force – both the origin of Ki and the place where it returns. The centre of the Hara is a point three finger widths below the navel, known as the Tanden or "Sea of Ki".

In Japan, to "have a good Hara" means to be in good health, to have vitality. To be "in Hara" means to be aware of yourself, coordinated and relaxed. The Hara is the centre of action, and to "move from your Hara" is the key to good shiatsu.

Keep the weight underside

The most important principle of shiatsu is to relax. Never hunch your back or raise your shoulders and always relax your elbows. Take the easy way and allow your Ki to work for you; it will, if you stay in your Hara. Relaxation connects you with the ground.

This principle, borrowed from Aikido, is a way of conveying the energy of the ground through your body. Whatever your position, imagine the upper side of your body or limbs are light and the lower aspects heavy – as though being pulled toward the earth. For example: when extending your arm to work with fingers, thumb, or palm, be aware of the heaviness of your elbow. Take energy from the earth up through your body. Lightly direct your Ki with your mind and let the earth provide both uplifting and pulling power. This is the essence of relaxed shiatsu.

Keeping your Hara open

You should aim to keep your Hara open when giving shiatsu, in all your movements. To do this, keep a wide base. Even when kneeling, keep a space at least the width of a fist between your knees. In this way your actions will flow more easily from the Tanden and you will keep in touch with the receiver's Ki. By keeping your centre of gravity in your Hara, you will also be able to work without losing your balance.

Visualizing circles

Ki is best conveyed along smooth open curves. Imagine a flexible sphere in front of your body, encompassed by your arms and chest, and smaller circles supporting your armpits, keeping all joints open and soft. These will help foster your Ki and at the same time keep your Hara open.

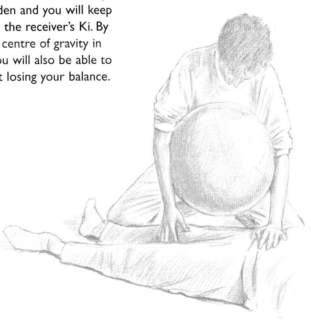

CHAPTER 7

AROMATHERAPY MASSAGE

Massage is used in aromatherapy both to assist the passage of essential oils into the body and to accentuate their therapeutic effects. Alone, massage can relax the muscles, enabling the blood and lymph to flow more freely, and soothe the mind. When these benefits are combined with the healing powers of essential oils, the results can be outstanding.

The two massage oil blends below nourish body and mind. The stimulating blend can help to improve poor circulation and will revive someone who is tired or run down. Keep the soothing blend for evening use, since it will relax the receiver and prepare her for sleep. Mix the essential oil with the carrier oils by shaking them well in a screw-topped bottle.

SOOTHING BLEND
2 drops Juniper Berry
3 drops Lavender
2 drops Sandalwood
15 ml (2.5 tsp) carrier oil

STIMULATING BLEND
3 drops Lemon
2 drops Rosemary
2 drops Juniper Berry
15 ml (2.5 tsp) carrier oil

To make your own blends, choose appropriate essential oils for your partner from the chart on page 250, making sure you observe any cautions and contraindications listed there. Prepare the oil according to the guidelines on page 29. Remember, never apply undiluted essential oils to the skin. Keep them away from the eyes. If you do get either neat or diluted essential oils in your eyes, rinse them immediately with plenty of clean water.

Before starting the massage, familiarize yourself with the basic strokes described on page 23. Prepare the room and yourself, following the guidelines on pages 28–30. Your partner should lie on a towel, to protect your working surface from the massage oil. You may also wish to use towels for privacy and warmth; notes in the sequence tell you when and where to position them.

Begin the massage by centring yourself (see page 30). You may also wish to use the cleansing visualization on page 30, or make the energy connection between you (see page 31).

Cautions

Citrus oils are photo-sensitive and may cause a skin reaction if exposed to ultraviolet light. Keep out of the sun for at least four hours after treatment with a citrus oil.

See page 5 for a full list of cautions and contraindications for massage.

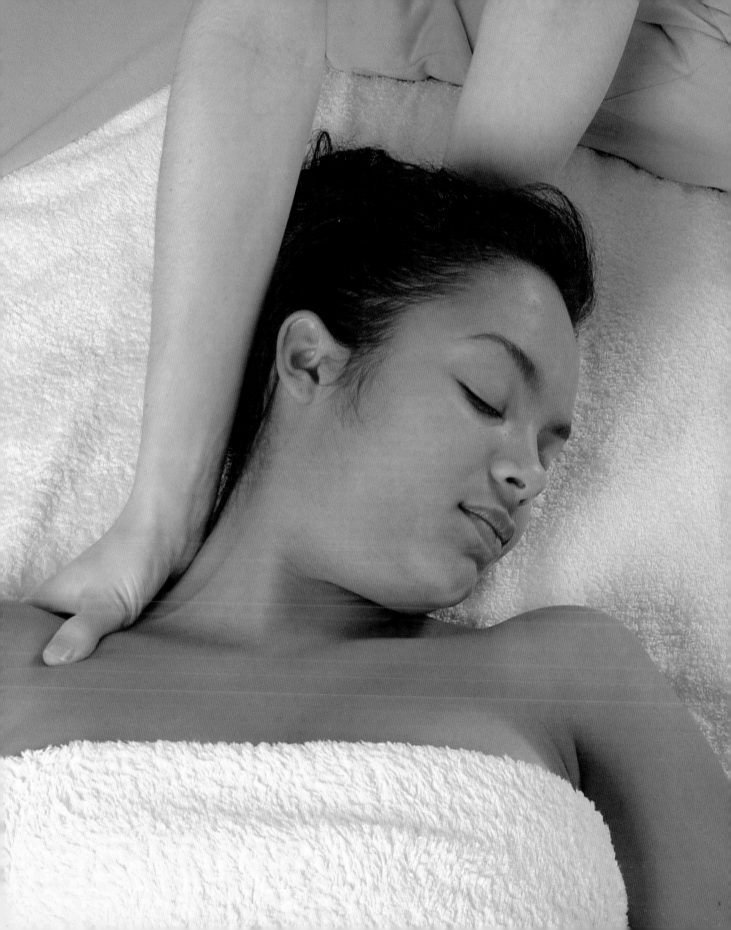

BACK

The receiver should lie on her front. A folded towel or pillow under her head, and a rolled towel under her ankles may make her more comfortable.

Spend a few quiet moments breathing deeply to release any tension. When you are fully relaxed, pour a little of the prepared blend of oils into your palm and rub your hands together briefly in order to warm the oil and distribute it evenly. During the massage, use a little more oil each time you move to work on a different part of the body.

If using towels, cover the buttocks and legs.

Step 1

Sit beside your partner at hip level, facing her head. Place your hands on the lower back, either side of the spine, with your fingertips pointing toward the shoulders. Slowly glide your hands up the back and out across the top of the shoulders, then down the sides of the body, returning to your starting point. Repeat, maintaining one continuous movement. A faster rhythm is more stimulating – a slower rhythm more relaxing. Repeat several times.

Step 2

Repeat the movement in step 1, but when you reach the shoulders stop to knead them. Work on one shoulder, then the other.

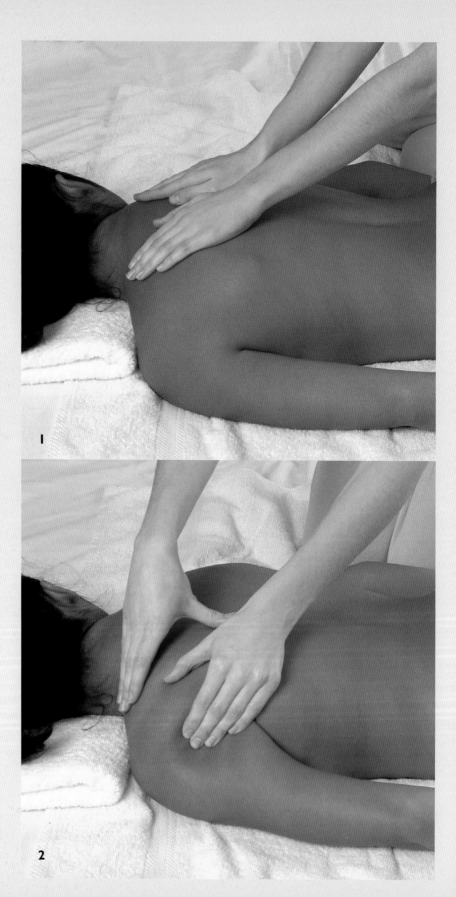

1

2

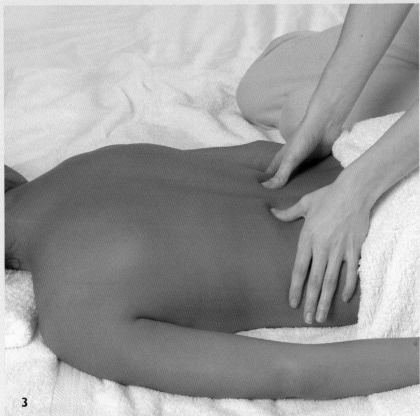

3

Step 3

Position your hands at waist level, with the pads of your thumbs in the hollows on either side of the spine, and your fingers open and relaxed. Push your thumbs firmly up the hollows for 5 cm (2 in), relax them, then move them back 2.5 cm (1 in). Continue in this way up to the neck. Then gently slide both hands back to the base of the spine. Repeat once more.

Repeat the first part of step 1, moving your hands up the back, round the shoulders and back down the sides of the body.

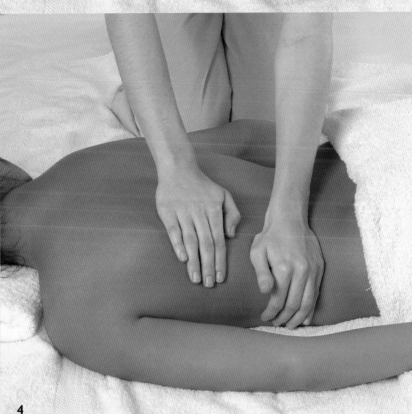

4

Step 4

Place one hand flat across the side of the back furthest from you, level with the base of the spine. Apply firm palm pressure, pushing away from you. Work up to the shoulders, using alternate hands. Repeat once more.

BACK

Step 5

Working on the side of the back furthest away from you, start with your hands at the top of the shoulder, lifting and squeezing the muscles that lie across this area. Roll the thumb of one hand toward the fingers of the opposite hand; repeat using alternate thumb and fingers. Continue this movement down the side of the body to the buttocks.

Move round to the other side of your partner and repeat steps 4 and 5 on the other side of the back. Finish by repeating the first part of step 1, moving your hands up the back, round the shoulders and back down the sides of the body.

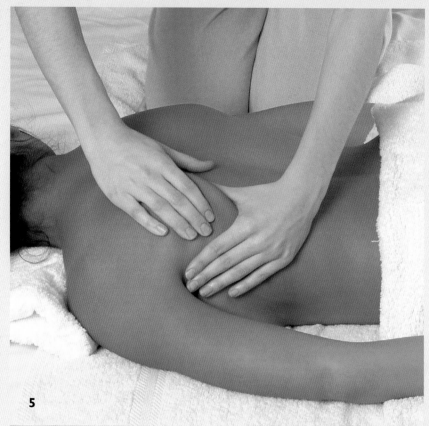

5

Step 6

Start with your thumbs at the base of the back, either side of the spine. Slowly work your way up the back, making tiny circles with your thumbs to focus the pressure. When you reach the shoulders, slide your hands down the back and repeat.

Caution: *Do not apply direct pressure to the spine.*

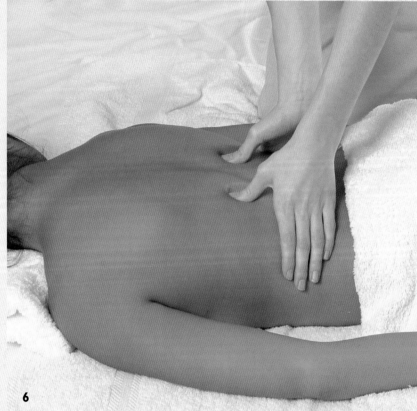

6

Step 7

Return your hands to the base of the spine, fingertips pointing toward the shoulders. Applying firm palm pressure up either side of the spine, work up to chest level. Then turn your fingers outward and apply palm pressure as you move your hands apart and outward to the sides of the body. Repeat this outward pressure movement at waist and hip levels.

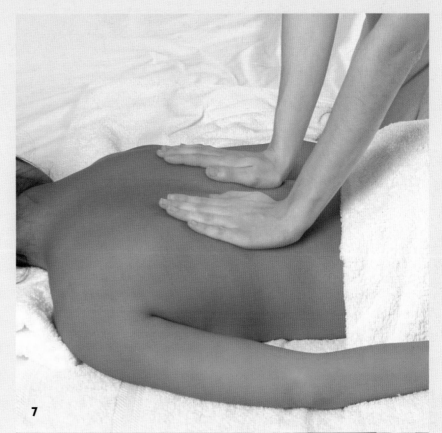

7

Step 8

Repeat the first part of step 1 again, moving your hands up the back, round the shoulders and back down the sides of the body.

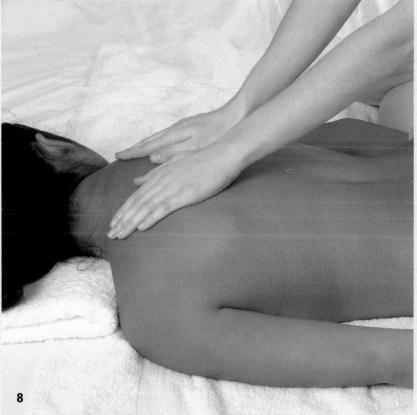

8

BACK OF LEGS AND FEET

If using towels, cover the back and shoulders.

Step 1

Move round to your partner's feet. Open your hands to form a "V" shape between your thumb and fingers. Then place your hands one below the other over the back of the ankle and glide up the leg. At the thigh, move one hand to each side of the leg and glide gently back down the sides. Repeat, gliding up and down in a continuous flow.

Caution: *Use only light pressure over the back of the knee.*

Step 2

Move to your partner's side and place your hands on the inside of the thigh. Roll the thumb of one hand toward the fingers of the opposite hand, then repeat using the opposite thumb and fingers. As thumb and fingers meet, the thigh muscles are lifted and squeezed. Continue this stroke, moving from the inner to the outer thigh. Repeat on the calf, lifting and squeezing the calf muscle.

Step 3

Move back to the feet. Slide the fingertips of both hands under the front of the ankle. Making tiny circles with your thumbs, apply pressure up either side of the tendon on the back of the ankle. Slide your thumbs down and repeat.

Caution: *Do not use this step on anyone who is pregnant.*

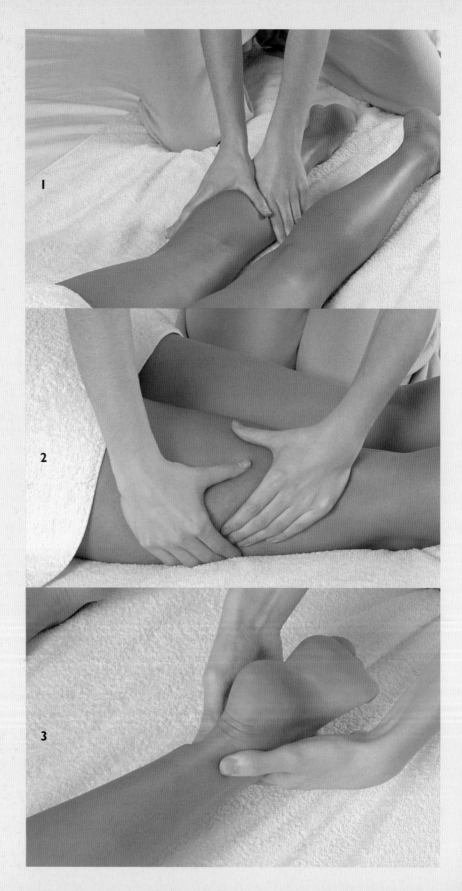

Step 4

Take the foot between your hands, so that the palm of your upper hand is resting in the arch. Pressing firmly and slowly, draw your hands down to the tip of the foot. Feet appreciate very firm pressure, and this "sandwich" stroke gives a wonderful feeling of wholeness when used with a leg massage.

Step 5

Hold the foot with your thumbs lying side by side on the sole, behind the toes. Pull both thumbs to the sides of the foot, then push them forward. Repeating this zig-zag movement, work gradually down to the heel. Then push firmly all the way back to the toes, keeping your thumbs side by side. Repeat the whole movement several times.

Repeat steps 1 to 5 on the other leg.

This completes the massage on the back of the body. After treating both legs, let your partner rest for a few moments. Then ask her to turn over for the massage on the front of the body. Arrange pillows and folded towels to make your partner comfortable.

If using towels, hold them up while your partner turns over.

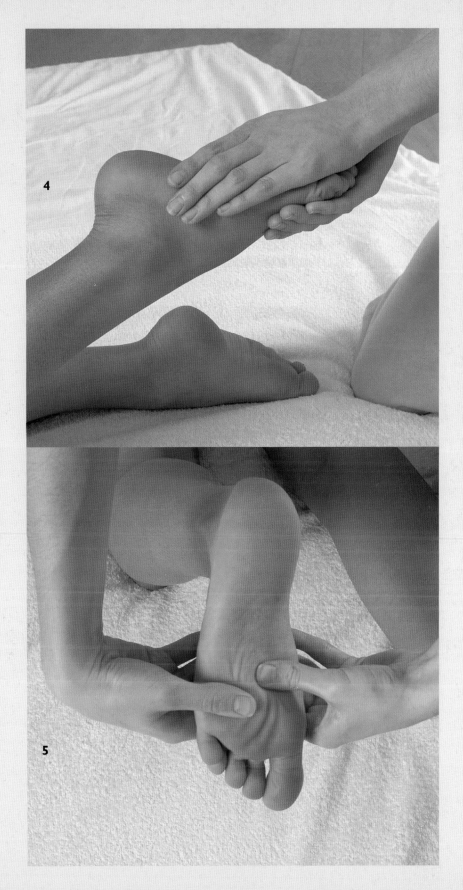

NECK AND HEAD

If using towels, cover the abdomen and legs.

Step 1
Move round to your partner's head and place your hands on the chest, fingertips pointing inward. Slide your hands apart across the shoulders, around the back of the shoulders, up the back of the neck, and behind the ears to the top of the head.

Caution: *Do not apply pressure on the front of the neck.*

Step 2
Slide your hands down the back of the neck. Starting at the base of the neck, use the tips of your middle three fingers to make small circles of pressure either side of the spine. Work slowly up the back of the neck and then outward along the base of the skull.

Step 3
Gently turn the head to one side. Working on the side away from the face, slide your hand down the side of the neck and cup the top of the shoulder in your palm. Apply gentle downward pressure to stretch the neck and shoulder. Repeat twice, then do the same on the other side.

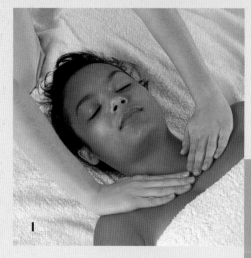

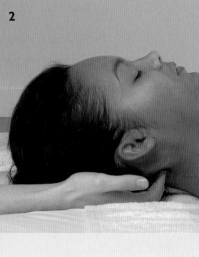

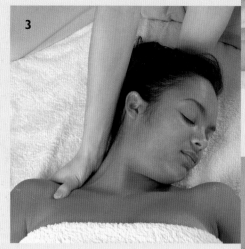

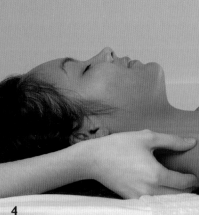

Step 4
Curl your fingers loosely and slide your hands under the base of the neck, so that your fingertips are on either side of the spine. Push firmly up into the muscle along the top of the shoulders, while moving your fingers back and forth individually. Continue this movement up the neck muscles until you reach the base of the skull. Relax and glide your hands smoothly back to the base of the neck. Repeat.

Step 5
Stroke up the side of the face, starting on the chin and working up to the forehead. Repeat several times, then finish by placing one palm across the forehead.

Step 6
Begin by stroking up the forehead with alternate palms. Then place the pads of the middle three fingers of both hands in the centre of the forehead between the eyes. Draw them gently apart across the brow and round the outside corner of the eyes. Use only your 4th fingers to return under the eyes toward the nose.

Step 7
Position your thumbs in the centre of the forehead. Using the three middle fingers of both hands, press firmly against the sides of the nose. Continue pressing along the top of the cheekbone until you reach the temple. Keeping your thumbs in position, return to the nose, pressing along the middle of the cheekbone.

Caution: *Do not use this step on anyone who has had surgery on the sinuses.*

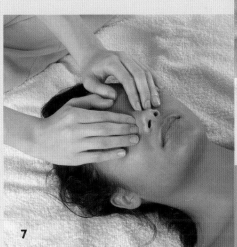
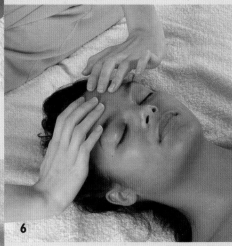
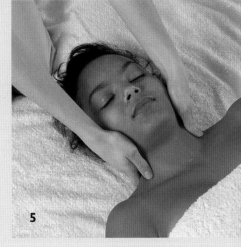
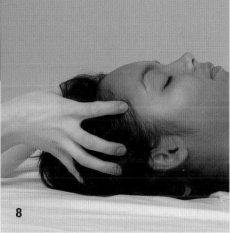

Step 8
Spread out your fingers and thumbs on both hands and place them on the scalp. Keep them in position and begin to move the scalp muscle over the bone by applying gentle pressure and circling slowly and firmly on the spot. Stop occasionally to move your hand position slightly, so you work gradually over the whole scalp.

CHEST AND ABDOMEN

If using towels, uncover the front of the torso.

Step 1

Move round to your partner's side. Place your palms on the midline of the chest, at the base of the ribcage. Slowly glide your palms up the chest, between the breasts and across the top of the shoulders, and back down the sides of the body to the starting position. Repeat in one continuous stroke, allowing your hands to mould to the contours.

Step 2

Imagine two semi-circles, one above and one below the navel. Place your left palm on the abdomen and use it to trace along each semi-circle in turn, in a clockwise direction. As your left hand moves away from you, place your right hand on the opposite side of the navel; let it trace the other semi-circle toward you, lifting it off the body to repeat. Maintain the stroke as one continuous movement.

Step 3

Position your thumbs on the lower border of the ribcage, either side of the midline. Ask your partner to take a deep breath in. On the out-breath, slowly slide your thumbs outward, with palms and fingers resting gently on the body. Repeat, making sure you only apply pressure on the out-breath. This stroke helps to "release" the diaphragm muscle.

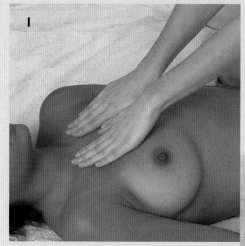

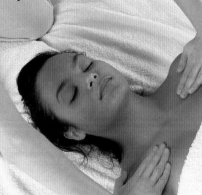

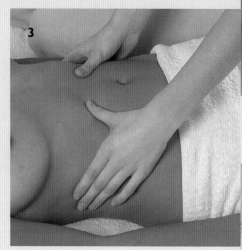

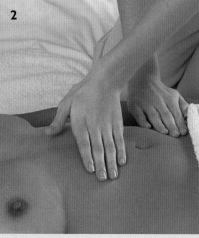

Step 4

Move round to your partner's head and place your hands on the chest just below the neck, fingers pointing inward. Move your hands slowly and firmly apart across the chest until the side of each palm is lying just above the underarm crease. Continue around the arms and along the shoulders to the back of the neck. Return with a light stroke to the chest. Repeat several times.

Step 5

Curl your fingers and place the middle sections in the centre of the chest. Draw your hands slowly apart toward the underarm crease. As you do so, begin knuckling by moving your fingers individually back and forth across the chest area. Return your hands smoothly to the centre of the chest, without applying pressure. Repeat.

Caution: *Do not use steps 6 to 8 on anyone who is pregnant.*

Step 6

Move to your partner's side again. Place the palm of one hand on the solar plexus, the soft area that lies directly beneath the breastbone. With the palm of your other hand, massage gently in a large circle, clockwise, around the navel, starting at the right side of the pubic bone. Work up that side of the abdomen, continue across the stomach, just below the other hand, and on down the abdomen to the starting point.

Step 7

Now place one hand on top of the other and, with your fingers relaxed, apply firm, even pressure with your palms as you move in small clock-wise circles around the abdomen, following the route in step 6.

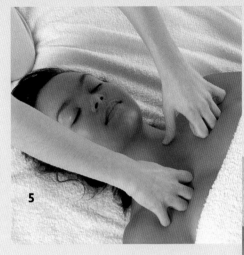

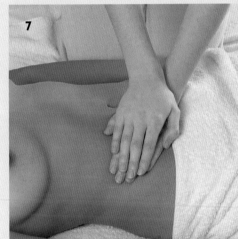

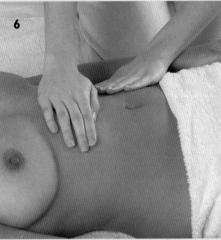

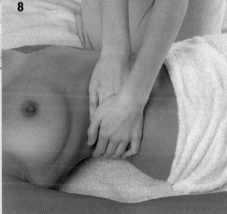

Step 8

Starting at hip level, on the side of the abdomen furthest from you, use alternate palms to lift the body toward its centre. Continue up to chest level. Repeat several times.

Bring one hand over to the near side of the abdomen and with the palm facing away from you, begin gently to lift this side of the abdomen. Follow with your other hand, and continue up to chest level using alternate hands.

165

ARMS AND HANDS

Work through steps 1 to 5 of this part of the sequence on one arm, then repeat on the other.

If using towels, cover the chest, abdomen, and legs.

Step 1
Holding your partner's hand, slowly glide your other hand up the arm, around the shoulder, and back down the arm. Swap hands and repeat, maintaining one continuous movement. You can raise the arm to enable the gliding hand to reach the underside of the limb.

Step 2
Bend your partner's elbow and rest the hand on the chest. Starting on the arm's inner surface, roll the thumb of one hand toward the fingers of the opposite hand. As thumb and fingers meet, the muscles of the inner arm are lifted and gently squeezed. Repeat using alternate thumb and fingers, moving from the inner to the outer arm.

Step 3
Hold your partner's wrist and gently raise the forearm. Place the thumb of your free hand just above the wrist and gently glide it up toward the elbow. Draw your hand back to the wrist and repeat, working up to the elbow in parallel lines. Although you are only applying pressure with your thumb, you should also keep the rest of your hand in gentle contact with the arm.

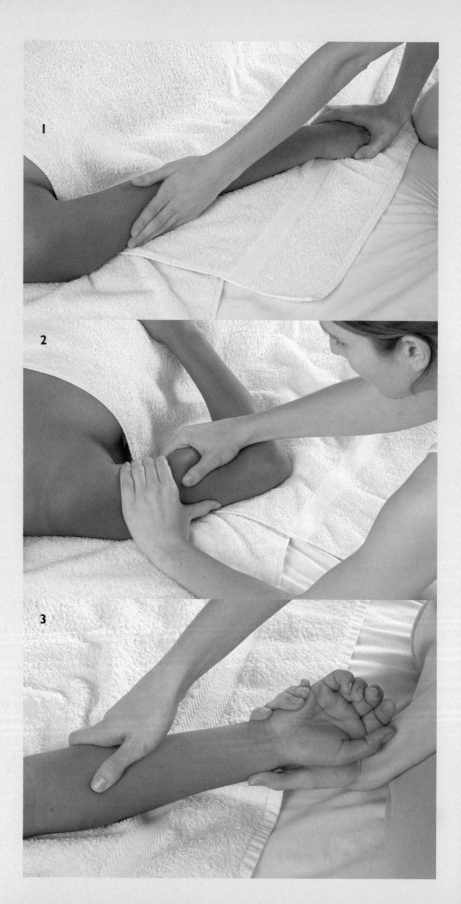

Step 4

Keeping the forearm raised, take hold of the hand as in a firm handshake. Gently place the palm of your free hand across the top of the wrist and close your fingers around it. Apply firm pressure and slide your hand up to the shoulder. Next slide your palm round underneath the arm and use a light stroke to return to the wrist. Repeat several times.

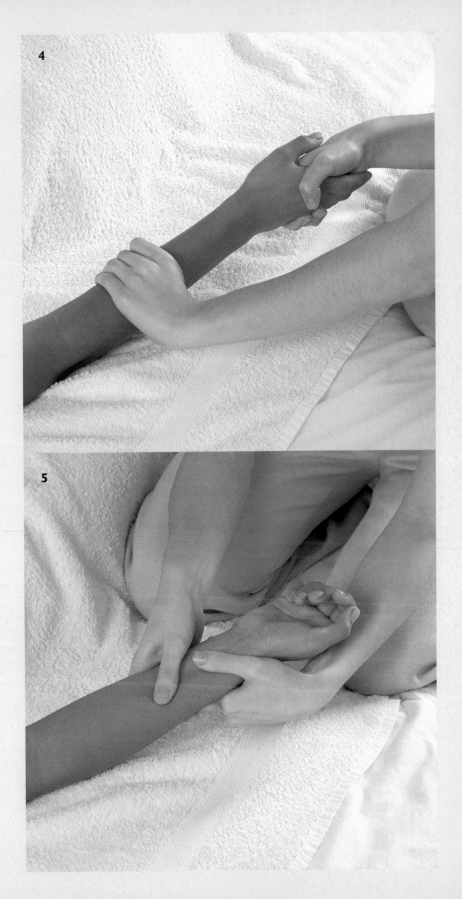

Step 5

Place your thumbs across the inside of the wrist, and apply pressure with both, in wide circles around the wrist area.

Then repeat step 4. As you finish, return the hand to your partner's side, holding it sandwiched between your palms. Relax your grip and pull off firmly.

Move to your partner's other side and repeat steps 1 to 5 on the other arm.

FRONT OF LEGS AND FEET

If using towels, cover the whole body, uncovering one leg at a time.

Step 1
Move to your partner's feet. Form a "V" shape between your thumb and fingers and place your hands one below the other over the front of the ankle. Glide up the leg. At the thigh, separate your hands and glide them gently back down the sides. Repeat, gliding up and down in a continuous flow.

Step 2
Placing your hands on either side of the thigh, bring the fingers of one hand toward the palm of the other, lifting and gently squeezing the large thigh muscle in between. Repeat over the whole of the upper leg.

Step 3
Starting at the ankle, place the heels of your hands on either side of the shin bone and move them in a circular motion. Work up to just below the knee, then slide your hands back and repeat.

Caution: *Do not use this step on anyone who is pregnant.*

Step 4
Firmly hold the top of the ankle, with your left hand for the right foot and vice versa, and use your other hand to circle the foot inward and toward the spine.

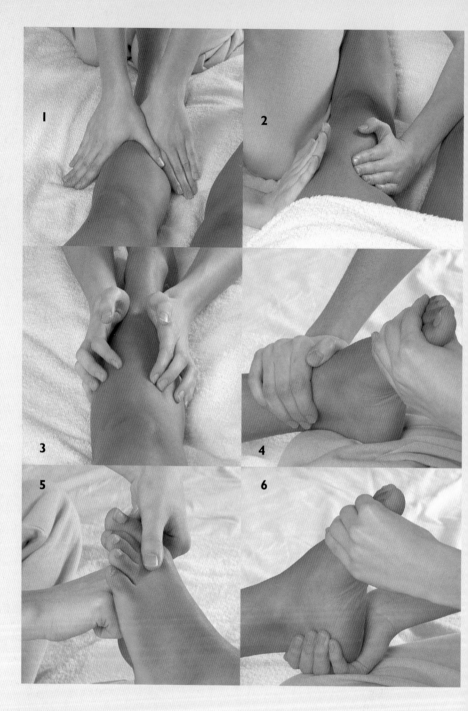

Step 5
Support the foot with toes pointing upward, with your fist behind the toes. Work the thumb of your other hand three times along the base of the first three toes.

Step 6
Slide your hand under the heel to support it, with your left hand for the right foot and vice versa, and use your other hand to circle the foot inward and toward the spine.

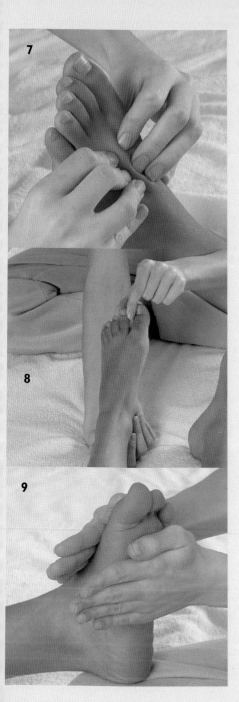

Step 7
Pressing into the sole of the foot with your thumbs, push across the top of the foot with the fingers of both hands simultaneously.

Step 8
Rest the heel in one hand. With the thumb and index finger of the other, pinch and knead the sides of each toe in turn.

Step 9
Holding the foot between your palms, rotate your hands around it in the motion of the wheels of a steam train.

CONNECTING

Now you have massaged each part of the body in turn, you need to connect the various parts to give your partner a sense of wholeness.

Move to your partner's side. Rest both your hands on the belly, then slowly (moving both hands simultaneously) glide one hand down one leg and off the foot and the other up to the opposite shoulder, down the arm, and off the hand. Bring the hands back to the belly and repeat the stroke along the other leg and arm.

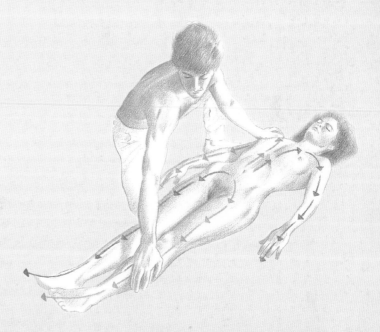

Cover your partner with a warmed towel and leave her to rest for a while. You may wish to use the clearing visualization, or break the energy connection between you (see page 31).

CHAPTER 8

REFLEXOLOGY

This reflexology sequence will improve the circulation and assist the body in speeding up the elimination of waste products, so that toxins do not have a chance to build up to harmful levels in the liver, kidneys, or bowel. It improves all of the body's functions and this in turn encourages the natural self-healing process to work more speedily and efficiently. A full foot session on a monthly basis, interspersed with occasional hand self-treatments (see pages 212–17), should be enough to maintain wellbeing.

Reflexology is easy to use in most environments and does not need any specialist equipment. The receiver should sit in a comfortable armchair, resting their legs on a low stool or chair and with their feet on a large cushion in the giver's lap. Use a foot moisturizer or balm – peppermint is particularly invigorating – to soften the feet, as this will make it easier for the giver to work over the feet with the thumb. If the foot is very dry, it will be harder to work the reflexes. However, only use a little moisturizer, and avoid using massage oil, as it is very hard to contact the reflexes properly on slippery skin.

This reflexology treatment takes about 45 minutes. Complete the entire sequence on the right foot first before treating the left. You treat the right foot first in order to work with the flow of the intestines: the intestine reflexes ascend on the right foot and descend on the left. The sequence ends with a winding-down massage for the neck, shoulders, and back. You can give this massage through clothes, or on bare skin using a little massage oil, with your partner either seated or lying down.

Before you start the massage sequence, familiarize yourself with the two basic strokes – creeping and rotating – described on page 25. Prepare yourself and the room, following the guidelines on pages 28–9. Begin the massage by sitting quietly for a few moments, and centre yourself using the meditation on page 30. You may also wish to use the cleansing visualization on page 30, and make the energy connection between you and your partner (see page 31).

The zones and reflexes used in the massage are shown clearly throughout the sequence. For more detail, refer to the reflexology foot maps on pages 246–7.

Caution: *See page 5 for a full list of cautions and contraindications for massage.*

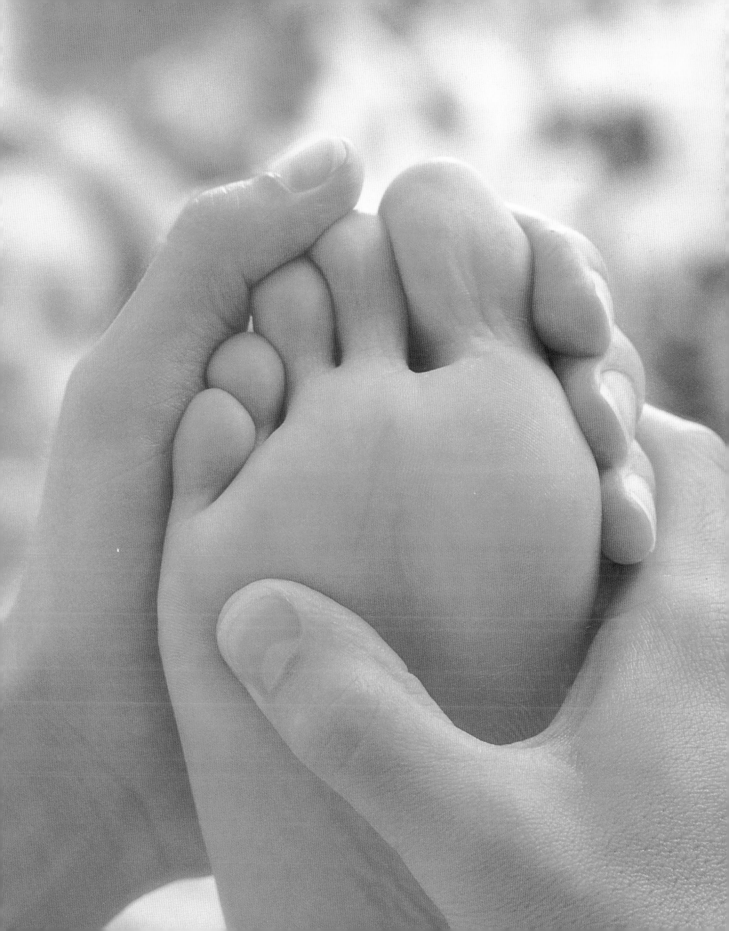

Before you begin, apply a little moisturizer to the foot.

Step 1
On the right foot, work along the diaphragm line, pressing with your thumb. This line runs across the foot along the top of the metatarsal bones where they meet the toes (see page 246). It is easy to identify, as the skin just above it is darker.

Caution: *Do not use this step on anyone who is pregnant.*

Step 2
Supporting the top of the foot, rock the whole foot from side to side between your palms, in a rapid but gentle movement.

Step 3
Support the ankle bones between the fleshy parts of your thumbs and rock the foot gently but rapidly from side to side, to free the ankle. Keep your wrists loose.

Step 4
For the right foot, push the fist of your right hand into the sole while squeezing the top of the foot with your left. This kneads the metatarsals, like kneading dough. Change hands when you work on the left foot.

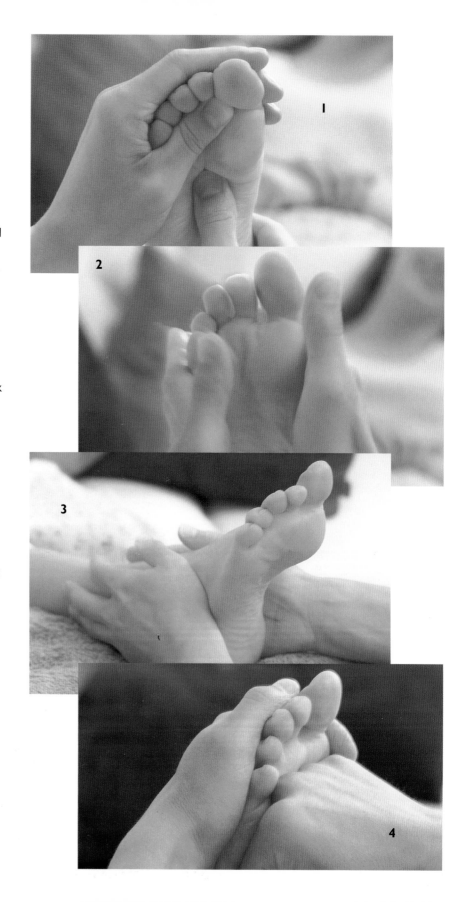

Step 5

Use the flat of your hand to rub vigorously up and down the inside of the foot. This stimulates and warms the spinal column.

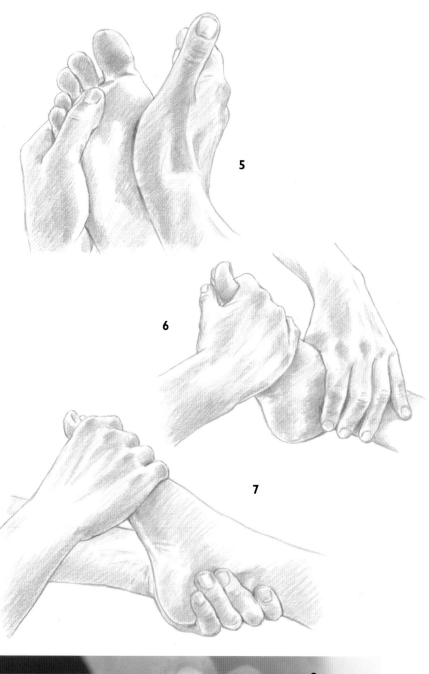

Step 6

For the right foot, firmly hold the top of the ankle with your left hand over the foot as shown, and circle the foot inward and toward the spine with your right.

For the left foot, hold the ankle with your right hand and circle the foot inward and toward the spine with your left. This exercise will help reduce swelling in the ankles.

Step 7

For the right foot, support the heel with your left hand underneath it as shown, and use your right hand to circle the foot gently inward and toward the spine. Reverse the hand positions for the left foot.

Step 8

Holding the foot between your two palms, rotate your hands around the foot, in a motion similar to the wheels on a steam train.

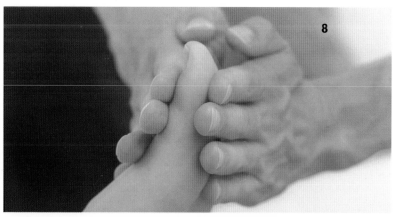

Step 9

Press into the sole of the foot with both your thumbs, and place your fingertips in line on either side of the top of the foot. Keeping your fingers flexed and the flat pads on your partner's foot, press down, then lift your fingers and slide forward a little and press again, in a creeping motion. This treatment relaxes the ribcage.

Step 10

Supporting the foot in an upright position, use the creeping technique with your thumb to work the lung reflex between the diaphragm line and shoulder line on the sole of the foot. Work upward, methodically, in parallel lines.

Step 11

Supporting the foot with your fist behind the toes, use your index finger to creep down the sinus reflexes in the grooves on the top of the foot.

Step 12

For the right foot, hold the top of the foot with your left hand and work with your right thumb; for the left foot, reverse the hand positions.

Starting at the base of the big toe, use the creeping technique to work up each toe in turn. Then change hands and work back along the toes again. This step works the sinus reflexes, and also the reflexes for the pineal gland, pituitary gland, hypothalamus, nose, and throat, on the big toe.

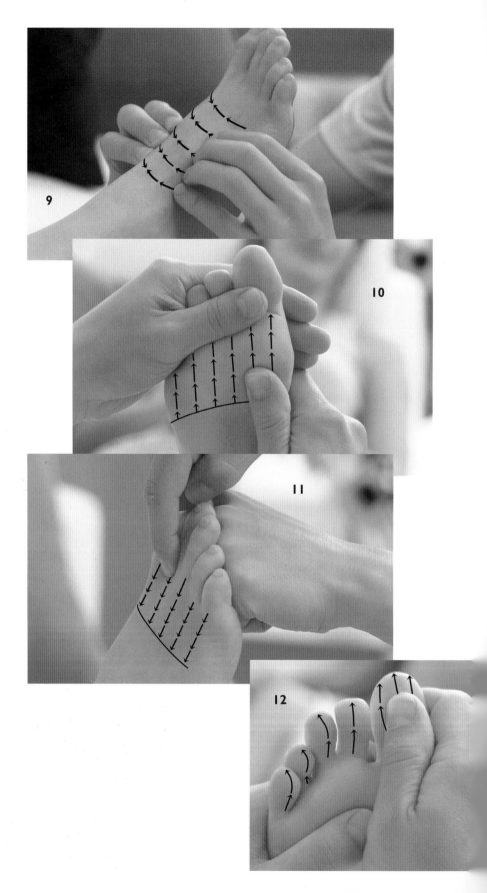

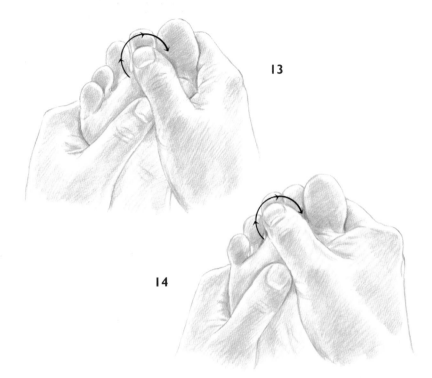

Step 13

For the right foot, support the top of the foot with your left hand and use your right thumb to work the eye reflex. For the left foot, reverse hand positions. Place the pad of your thumb under the first bend of the second toe and rotate it inward, toward the spine, using a small but firm movement. Maintain the pressure for several seconds for maximum benefit.

Step 14

Still supporting the top of the foot, work the ear reflex under the first bend on the third toe, using thumb rotations.

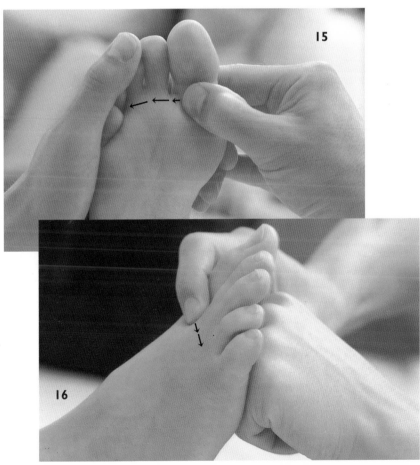

Step 15

With your thumb, use a creeping motion in a line along the base of the first three toes, starting at the big toe. Repeat three times. This treats the neck and thyroid reflexes on the sole.

Step 16

Supporting the foot with your fist behind the toes, use your index finger to creep along the base of the first three toes on the top of the foot, starting at the big toe. Repeat three times to treat the neck and thyroid reflexes on the top of the foot.

Step 17

To work the coccyx on the right foot, hold the top of the foot with your right hand and creep up the inside of the heel with the four fingers of your left hand, as shown.

For the hip and pelvis, swap hand positions and creep up the outside of the heel with the fingers of your right hand. Reverse the hand positions for the left foot.

Step 18

On the right foot, use your right thumb to creep up the spine reflex on the inside edge of the foot to the top of the big toe. Use your left thumb for the left foot.

Step 19

Use your index finger to creep up the edge of the big toe to treat the cervical spine reflex.

Step 20

To treat the neck, work down the other edges of the first three toes, using your thumb and a creeping motion. Use your right thumb on the right foot, and vice versa.

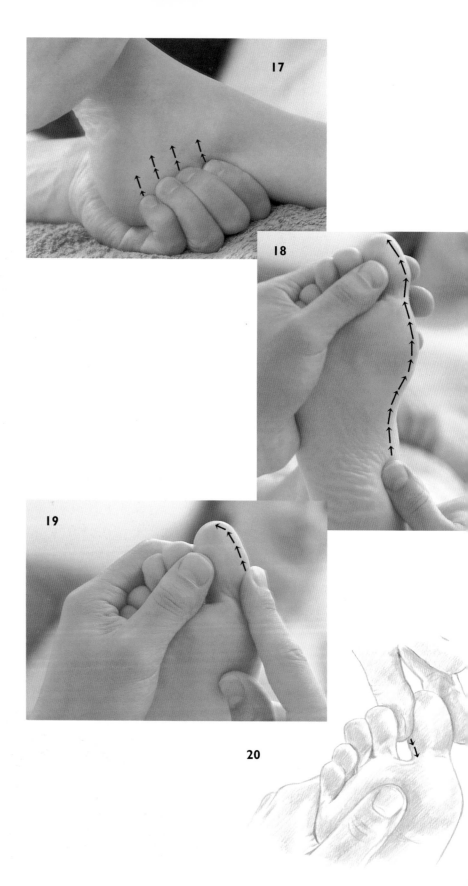

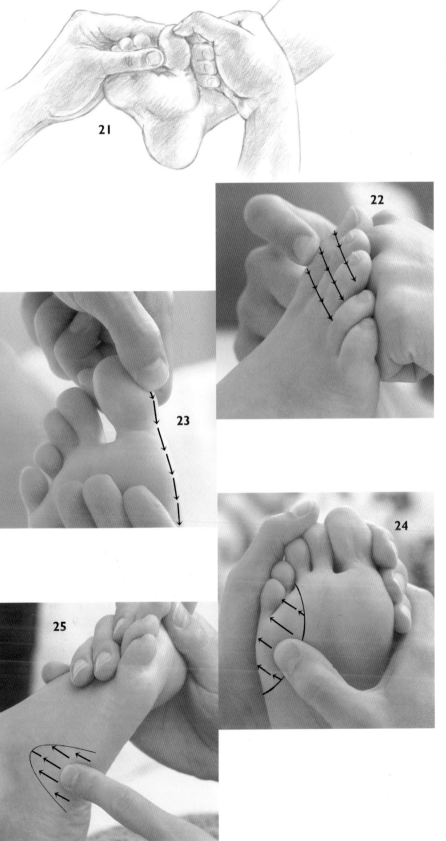

Step 21

Supporting the right foot with your left hand, work over the top of the big toe with your right thumb, using a creeping motion. This contacts the brain reflex. Reverse the hand positions for the left foot.

Step 22

Support the right foot with your left fist behind the toes. Use your right index finger to creep along the face reflex on the first three toes. Change hands for the left foot.

Step 23

Supporting the sole with the back of your non-working hand, use your thumb to creep down the inside edge of the foot, working the spine reflex.

Step 24

Cradling the top of the foot, creep your thumb outward in parallel lines across the shoulder area between the two smallest toes, as shown. Change hands and creep inward along these lines with your other thumb.

Step 25

Creep your index finger in parallel lines across the triangular-shaped reflex for the knee and elbow, on the outside of the foot.

Step 26

Use your index finger to creep up the primary sciatic area behind the ankle bone, continuing about 4 cm (1.5 in) up the leg.

Step 27

The secondary sciatic area lies across the heel on the sole of the foot, halfway between the pelvic line (see p. 246) and the bottom of the foot. Creep along this line two or three times with your thumb, starting at the inside edge of the foot each time.

Steps 28 to 30 are for the right foot only. Omit these steps when following the sequence for the left foot.

Step 28

The liver reflex is on the right foot only. Support the foot with your left hand and creep your right thumb across, from the inside to the outside in parallel diagonal lines (A). Change hands and work in the opposite direction (B).

Step 29

The ileocecal valve joins the large and small intestines, and its reflex is on the outside of the right foot, near the pelvic line. Press down firmly on this point with your left thumb and then use the flat of your thumb to make an outward-hooking movement in the shape of the letter "J". Working this point improves bowel function.

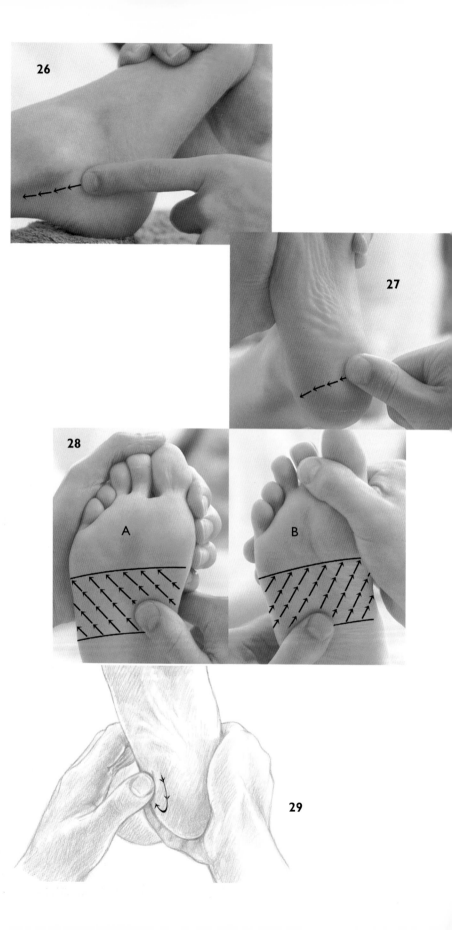

Step 30

These reflexes for the ileocecal valve, ascending and transverse colon, and small intestines are on the right foot only. Support the right foot with the left hand and use your right thumb to work the area under the waist line on the sole (see p. 246), in parallel lines starting at the inside of the foot (A). Swap hands and work back across in the opposite direction (B).

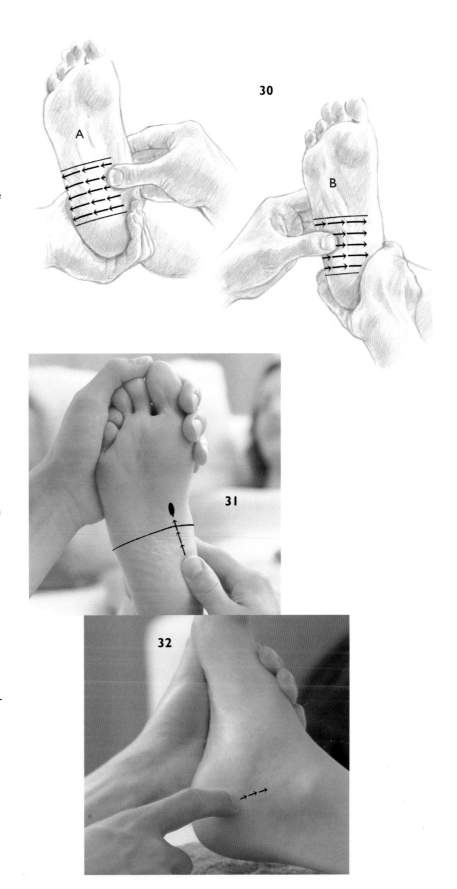

Step 31

To contact the bladder and ureter tube, creep up the inside edge of the ligament line to the waist line. The kidney and adrenal reflexes lie above the intersection of the waist and ligament lines (see p. 246). Place the flat pad of your thumb on this point and rotate it inward, toward the spine, using a small but firm movement. Maintain the pressure for several seconds.

Step 32

Support the right foot in your left hand and use your right index finger to creep from the tip of the heel to the inside ankle bone. The reflex point for the uterus/prostate is halfway along this line. For the left foot, reverse the hand positions.

Step 33

Press in with your two thumbs on the sole of the foot, while you use the first two fingers of both hands to creep across the top of the foot between the ankle bones, along the fallopian tube/vas deferens reflex, to meet in the middle. Repeat two or three times.

Step 34

Support the right foot in your right hand and use your left index finger to creep from the tip of the heel to the outside ankle bone. The reflex point for the ovary/testis is halfway along this line. For the left foot, reverse the hand positions.

Caution: *Do not use this step on anyone who is pregnant.*

Now repeat steps 1 to 27 and 31 to 34 on the left foot, before following steps 35 to 38 on the left foot only.

Step 35

The main reflex for the heart is a rectangular shaped reflex that sits on the diaphragm line beneath the first three toes and finishes halfway between the diaphragm and shoulder lines, on the left foot. Do not treat this area more than three times, as you have already worked it when contacting the lung reflex in step 10. (The reflexes overlap, just as the organs do in the body.) Support the top of the left foot with your right hand, and creep your left thumb across from the big toe to the third toe. Repeat step 1 (page 172) to relax the diaphragm.

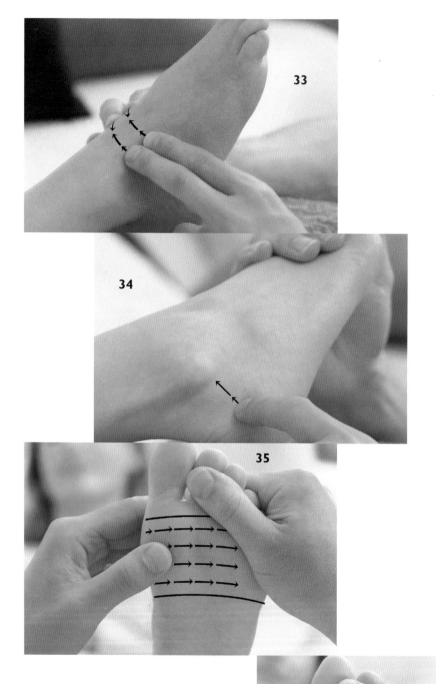

Step 36

The main stomach reflex is on the left foot, between the diaphragm and waist lines. Support the foot with your right hand and use your left thumb to creep across the area in diagonal parallel lines, as shown. Change hands and work diagonal lines in the opposite direction, with your right thumb.

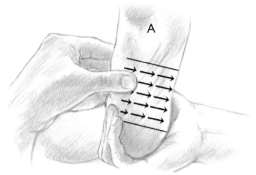

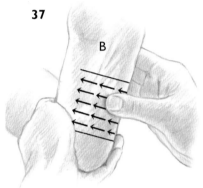

37

Step 37

The intestine reflexes on the left foot are for the small intestines, the transverse descending colon, and the sigmoid colon.

Support the heel with your right hand and use your left thumb to creep across the area under the waist line in parallel lines, starting at the inside edge (A). Change hands and repeat, working in the opposite direction (B).

WINDING-DOWN MASSAGE

The receiver can sit or lie, as preferred. The massage can be given through clothing, or on bare skin using massage oil.

Step 1

If you are using massage oil, apply a little to your palms. Use slow, circular movements to massage across your partner's shoulders and up either side of the spine. Use the tips of your fingers to work up the back of the neck with gentle rotations or kneading.

Step 2

Start with your palms at either side of the base of the spine, and work up both sides to the neck, with circular movements. Repeat four times.

Step 3

Return to the base of the spine and work up either side of it again, making small circular movements with the tips of your index fingers. Repeat. Finish by sliding your palms up either side of the spine and out across the shoulders.

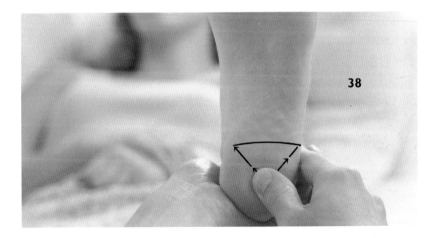

38

Step 38

The "V"-shaped sigmoid colon reflex is found under the pelvic line, on the left foot only. Cup the base of the heel in your right hand and

use your left thumb to creep up the right-hand fork of the "V". Then swap hands and use your right thumb to creep up the left-hand fork.

Leave your partner to rest for a while. You may wish to use the clearing visualization, or break the energy connection between you (see page 31).

CHAPTER 9

HEAD MASSAGE

Head massage tones the muscles and releases stress and tension. By stimulating the body's energy channels and pressure points (see page 15) the massage also balances energy in the internal organs, while stimulation of the lymphatic system boosts immunity, and of the endocrine system balances the hormones. It also affects the pulsing rhythms of the cerebrospinal fluid, carrying healing messages around the body and stimulating the body's self healing mechanisms. Tension in the muscles is released, dispersing toxins, reducing mental and physical stress, and improving blood flow to the brain.

Given regularly, preferably once a week, the massage also has a cumulative beneficial effect on your mental state. Relaxation frees up your creativity, so you can deal with day-to-day problems and challenges more easily.

Traditional Indian head massage is usually given with the receiver seated. However, some people prefer to be massaged lying down. You should choose whichever feels more comfortable for you and your partner. The step-by-step instructions assume your partner is seated, but you can adapt them to a lying position.

Whichever position your partner chooses, you need to be relaxed and comfortable in order to guide him or her into deep relaxation. If you need to change position during the treatment, move slowly and rhythmically so your partner is unaware of any break. To work with your partner seated, select a chair that is high enough for you to reach the scalp and shoulders without bending. Your partner should sit with feet flat on the floor, hands in the lap, and shoulders back. You should stand squarely behind your partner, wearing comfortable shoes or with bare feet, and maintain a straight posture.

This massage sequence takes 30–40 minutes. After massaging your partner you may wish to wait 15–20 minutes to ground yourselves before swapping roles. Before you start, prepare the room and yourself (see pages 28–9) and familiarize yourself with the basic head massage techniques described on pages 26–7. Begin the massage by centring yourself and use the cleansing meditation if you wish (see page 30). The massage starts with vigorous work on the shoulders and upper back, before moving on to the slower and more meditative head massage.

Caution: *See page 5 for a full list of cautions and contraindications for massage.*

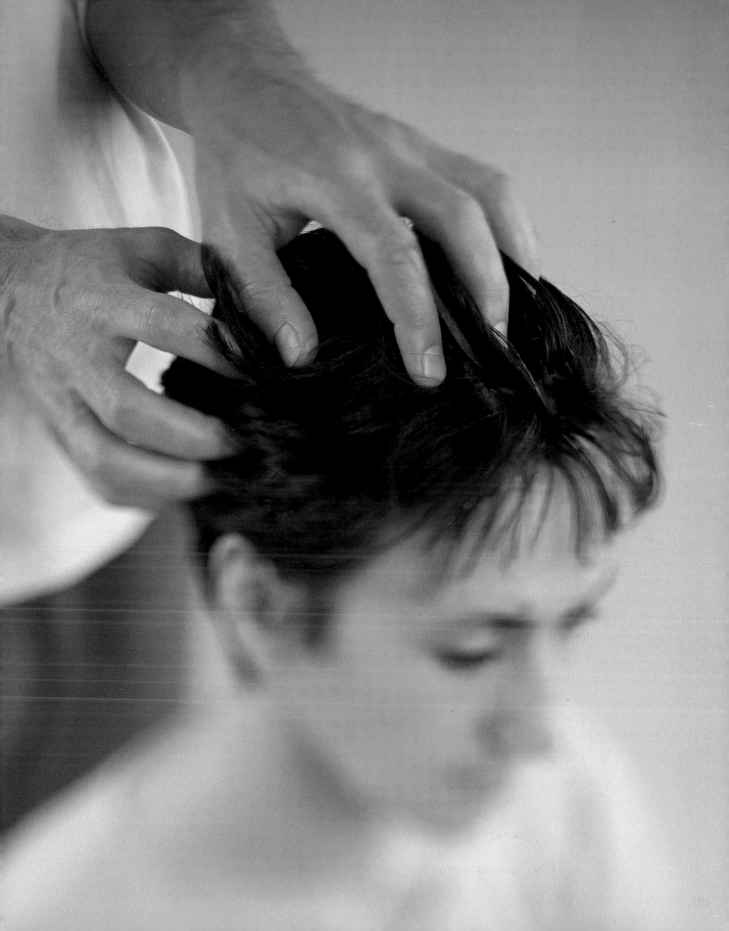

UPPER BACK AND SHOULDERS

Step 1

Position the heels of your hands on either side of your partner's spine, level with the bottom of the shoulder blades. Lean your body weight on to your hands, pushing the muscles outward. Then creep hand over hand up the back, parallel to the spine, to the base of the neck, keeping your hands always in contact with the back. Repeat two or three times to loosen the tension in the upper back.

Caution: *Do not apply strong pressure directly on the spine.*

Step 2

Place the pads of your thumbs either side of the spine, level with the lower edge of the shoulder blades. Leaning strongly on to your thumbs, rotate firmly for 3–5 seconds. Then move your thumbs out two finger widths and repeat, working along a horizontal line to the edge of the back. Start the next horizontal line beside the spine, two finger widths up from the first, and continue in this way up the back until you reach the neck.

Step 3

Use thumb rotations with downward pressure at two finger width intervals across the tops of the shoulders.

Caution: *Do not massage the midpoint of the shoulders on anyone who is pregnant.*

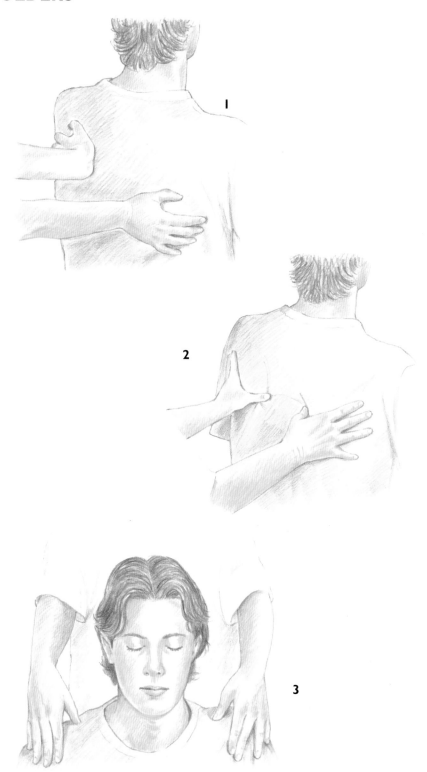

Step 4

Starting with the heels of your hands either side of the spine and level with the bottom of the shoulder blades, lean and roll in across the heels, at the same time pushing the muscles outward. Work across the back in lines, up to the base of the neck, as in step 2.

4

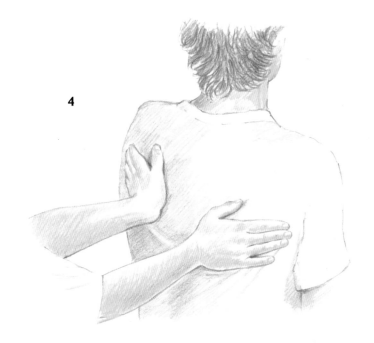

Step 5

5

Clench your hands into fists and use strong pressure and a rolling action to knuckle up the upper back, pushing the muscles outward from the spine. You can work hand over hand all over one side and then the other, or else use both hands simultaneously to work in lines out from the spine over the whole upper back, as in step 2.

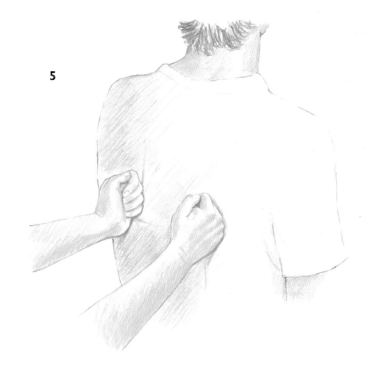

SHOULDERS AND ARMS

Caution: *Do not massage the midpoint of the shoulders of anyone who is pregnant.*

Step 1

Place the backs of your forearms at the base of your partner's neck, on either side of the head. Your hands should face upward, fists loosely clenched. Lean down strongly for a count of five.

Now rock your body back, move your arms four finger widths away from the neck, and lean down again. Repeat this action across the tops of the shoulders until you reach the tops of the arms.

Step 2

From your position in step 1, rotate your forearms inward so your fists face each other. Keeping a strong pressure, slide your forearms down the outside of your partner's arms to the elbows. Repeat twice more, then rub all over the arms, back, and shoulders.

Step 3

Grasp your partner's shoulders either side of the neck. By pushing down with the heel of your hand and pulling with your fingers, pinch (don't nip) the flesh of the shoulders in a forward, rolling motion. The heels of your hands should slide toward your fingertips. Move your hands about a palm's width out across the shoulders and repeat, working down the arms to the hands. If you cannot reach both arms at once, treat one at a time, with a two-handed wringing action.

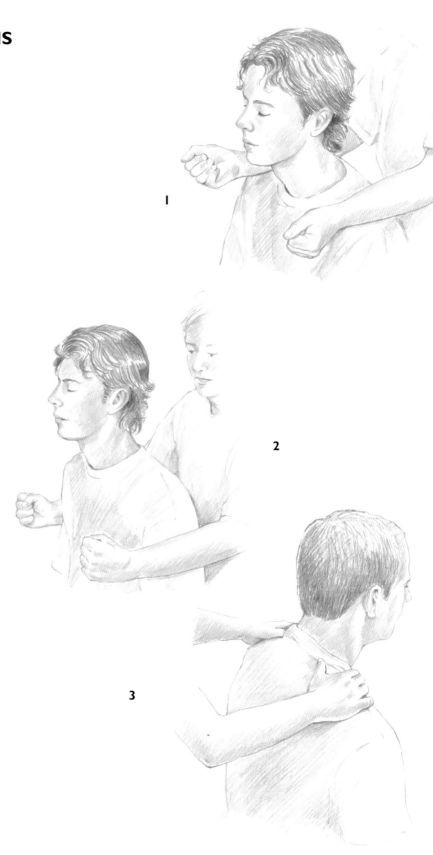

Step 4

Place your elbows at the base of your partner's neck, either side of the head, with your forearms extended in front of you, palms facing upward, and fists lightly clenched. Close your fists and lean your body weight gently on to your elbows, bringing your fists up toward you slowly. The closer you bring your fists toward you, the sharper your elbows and the greater the pressure. Rotate your elbows for a count of five.

Relax and move your elbows about three finger widths toward the arms and repeat, until you have covered the whole of the shoulders.

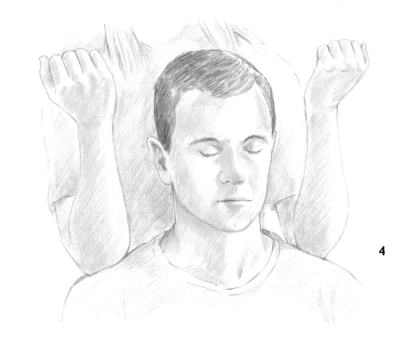

Step 5

Return your elbows to the base of your partner's neck, about four finger widths either side of the spine. Repeat the movement from step 4, working down your partner's back as far as you can.

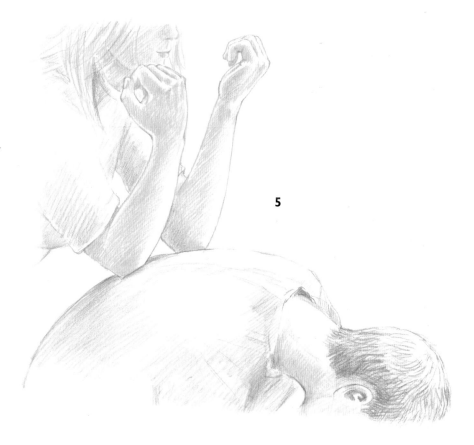

NECK

Caution: *Do not use steps 1 and 2 on anyone with a medical neck condition.*

Step 1

Place your hands on the shoulders, with your thumbs either side of the spine at the base of the neck. Leaning your weight on to your thumbs, use thumb rotations to work up the neck on both sides of the spine two finger widths from the midline, until you reach the base of the skull. Keep the pressure firm and even. Repeat twice more.

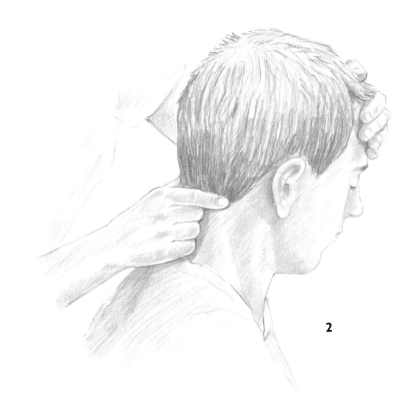

1

Step 2

Support the forehead with one hand, allowing the head to drop forward slightly. Place the four fingers of your other hand in line about a finger width to the right and parallel to the spine. Gently rotate your fingertips for a count of ten, in a slow, flowing movement. Repeat the movement three times, working your fingers out away from the spine. Change hands and repeat on the other side of the spine.

Now place your first finger and thumb either side of the spine, close to the head, in the hollows where the vertebrae meet the skull. Press strongly in an upward direction into these points for a count of five, then relax.

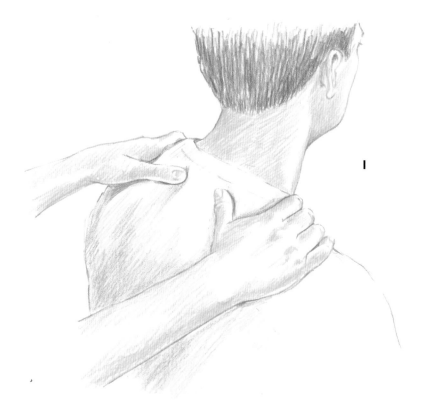

2

HEAD

Caution: *Do not use firm pressure on the top of the head on the very young, the elderly, or anyone with epilepsy, bone disease, or clinical depression.*

Step 1
Hold your partner's head lightly, with your hands on the sides, until your breathing synchronizes. This steadying action prepares you both for the more relaxing part of the massage routine. As you hold the position, visualize a clear, bright light from far above you, passing through your body into your partner's body, and down into the earth.

Step 2
Stroke lightly all over your partner's hair with the palms of your hands. Then comb through the hair loosely with your fingers apart and relaxed, separating the hair but not touching the scalp. These soothing movements keep a smooth, flowing rhythm as you change from one technique to another.

Step 3
With your hands on either side of the neck, slide them up into the hair, fingers apart, keeping close to the scalp. When you have gathered a handful of hair, close your fingers firmly and pull away from the head. Allow the hair to move through your fingers under tension, creating a strong, even pull. Repeat all over the head, always pulling the hair at right angles away from the scalp.

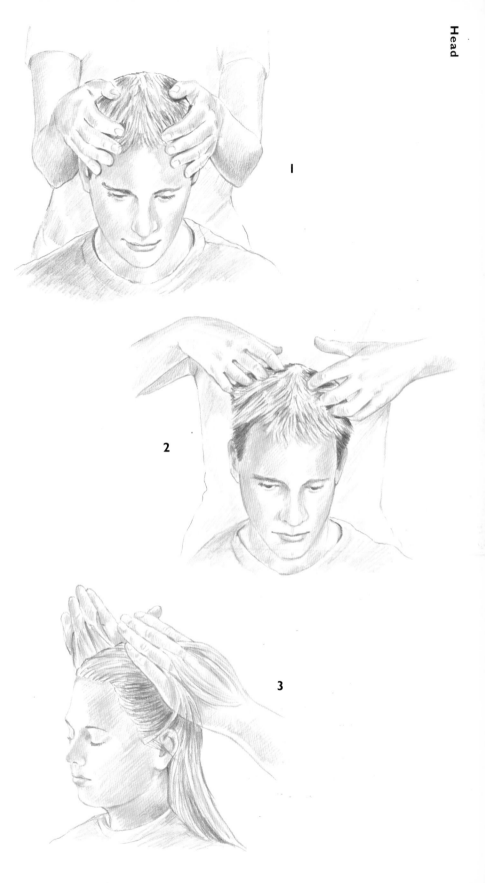

HEAD

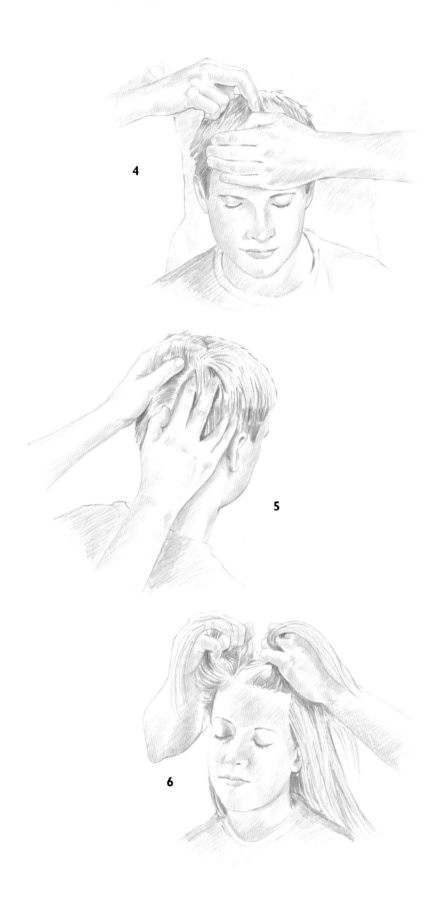

Step 4

Support the forehead with one hand, and use two fingers of the other hand to make rotations from the hairline back along the midline at one finger width intervals. Work over the top of the head and down to the base of the skull. Here press upward with both fingers for a count of three. Return to the hairline and work a parallel line two finger widths from the first line. Finish by pressing upward at the base of the skull for a count of three. Continue until you have covered one side of the head. Stroke the hair for a few seconds, then change hands and repeat on the other side of the head.

Step 5

Starting at the base of the skull, stroke and comb up through the hair toward the hairline, working over the scalp in the opposite direction to the rotations in step 4.

Step 6

Run both your hands up into the hair over the top of the head. When you have collected a handful, hold firmly and lightly shake the scalp back and forth. Don't pull hard – just enough to move the scalp.

Step 7

Hold your fingers with your nails in line and lightly scratch all over the head, keeping your wrists loose. Stroke or comb through the hair for a few moments.

Caution: *Do not work on broken skin, or sore areas of the scalp.*

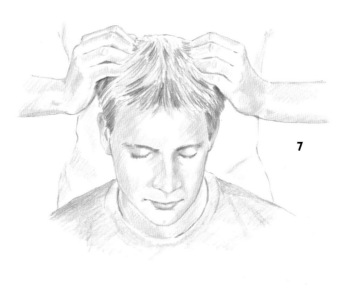

Step 8

Support the forehead with one hand, and use one finger of the other hand to apply pressure for 3–5 seconds at one finger width intervals along the midline. Start at the hairline and work back over the head to the nape of the neck. Work over the side of the head in the same way, in parallel lines two finger widths apart. Stroke the hair lightly and change hands to work on the other side of the head. This technique is excellent for "heavy" headaches, tension, and eye strain.

Stroke or comb through the hair again, from the nape of the neck to the hairline.

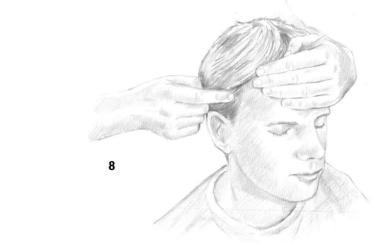

Step 9

Hold your hands so your fingertips are level. Keeping your wrists loose, and with both hands tapping together, bounce your fingertips off the hair with quick, light, smooth movements and a regular rhythm. Move over the head in lines, starting at the hairline and working back to the nape of the neck, then continuing out over the shoulders in a swift sweep.

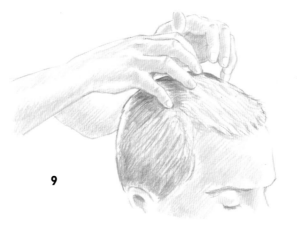

HEAD

Step 10

Beat with the side of each hand alternately in a light chopping action all over the head, neck, upper back, and shoulders, keeping a regular rhythm.

Step 11

Support the forehead with one hand. Make a fist with the other and place your knuckles on the back of the neck. Rock your fist against the neck, from the little finger to the index finger and back again, applying firm and steady pressure. In this way, knuckle up the neck and back of the head in a vertical line, then work a parallel line, two finger widths from the first, over the side of the head. Stroke all over the hair, then change hands and repeat on the other side.

Step 12

Support the forehead with one hand. Place the heel of the other at the nape of the neck and knead, by applying strong pressure while rolling from the heel up over the palm to the fingertips. Knead up the back of the neck and head to the crown, then start again at the nape and knead up the side of the head.

Stroke all over the hair, then change hands and repeat on the other side. Then knead the top of the head, from crown to forehead.

Rub all over the head briskly, then gently comb or stroke the hair.

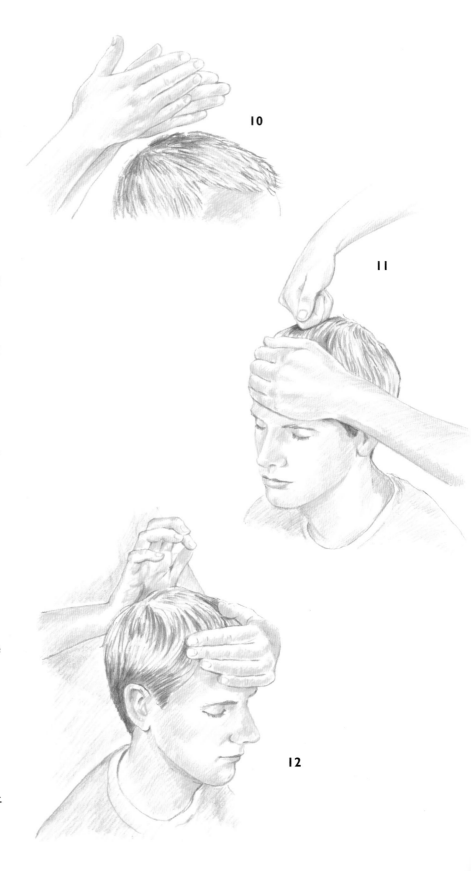

10

11

12

192

FACE

Caution: *Do not massage the lymphatic areas on the sides of the face, the throat, across the chin, or behind the ears of anyone who has cancer.*

Do not massage the throat of anyone who is pregnant.

Step 1

Allow your partner's head to rest against you. With the fingertips of both hands meeting under the chin, lightly stroke upward and outward. Move your hands to meet under the nose and stroke again. Then move your hands to meet on the nose and, avoiding the eyes, stroke again. Finally place your hands so they meet on the forehead and stroke outward and upward again. Repeat three or four times.

Step 2

Use your fingers to stroke up the throat and round under the ears, using alternate hands and brisk, light movements, for about 30 seconds.

Step 3

Place your fingertips in line across the centre of the forehead. Ask your partner to tense the muscles under your fingertips for a count of ten, then release. Move your hands two finger widths apart and repeat, working across the forehead.

Move your hands down so that your fingertips are in line across the middle of the nose and repeat the tensing and releasing, until you reach the ears. Move down again to cover the area from the nose to the chin.

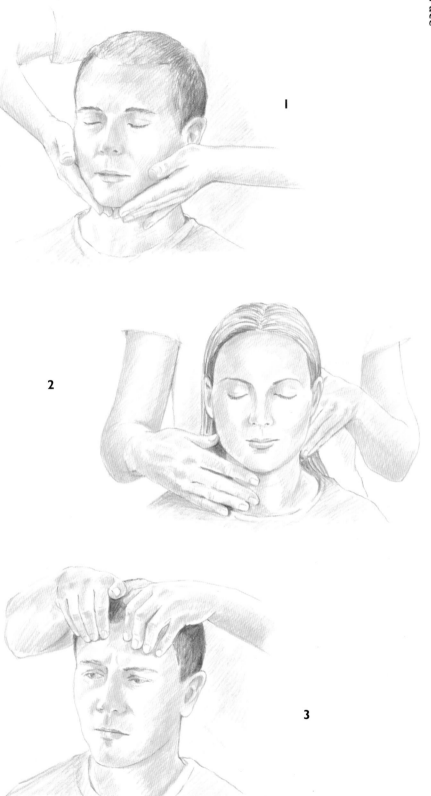

1

2

3

FACE

Step 4

With light, brisk finger movements, stroke up the sides of the face from the jaw to the temples. Place the fingertips of each hand in a vertical line in the middle of the forehead, and rotate your fingertips, applying firm pressure, for 3–5 seconds. Move your hands apart two finger widths and repeat, until you have covered the whole forehead.

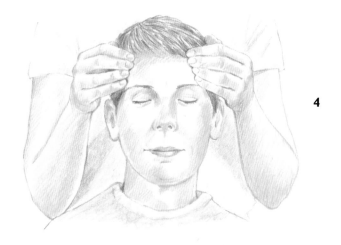

4

Step 5

Starting with your index fingers side by side in the middle of the chin, rotate your fingertips, applying firm pressure for 3–5 seconds. Move your fingers one finger width apart and repeat, working along the jawbone. Repeat in parallel lines at two finger width intervals up over the cheeks, finishing on the cheekbones. Now apply firm pressure with two fingers of each hand under the middle of the chin for 3–5 seconds. Repeat along the jawbone, moving two finger widths each time.

5

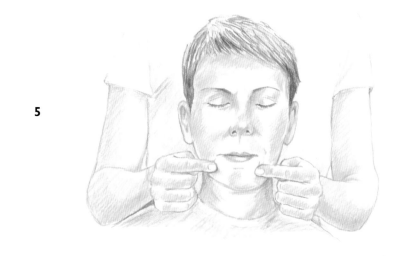

Step 6

Use one or two fingers to knead along the lower gums, starting in the middle of the jaw and moving outward and back. Knead for 3–5 seconds in each position, before moving two finger widths to the next. Then repeat along the upper gums. This technique stimulates blood flow to the gums and encourages healthy teeth.

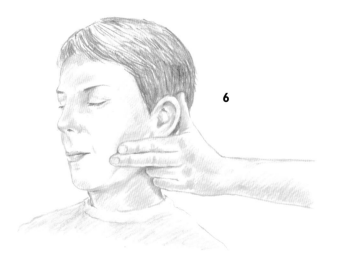

6

EARS

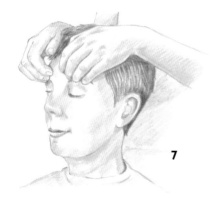

Step 1
Hold the tops of the ears, close to the head, between finger and thumb. Rub firmly down around the outer edge of the ear (A). Hold the lobes and pull down for a count of ten (B). Then return to the top of the ears, move one finger width into the "shells" of the ear, and repeat the rubbing and pull on the lobes. Repeat until you have massaged all the nooks and crannies of the ear.

Rub the ears briskly with your palms, then cup your hands over them for 3–5 seconds. They will probably be quite hot and your partner may hear a buzzing sound for a few moments.

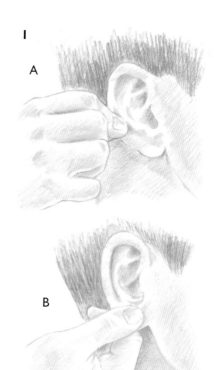

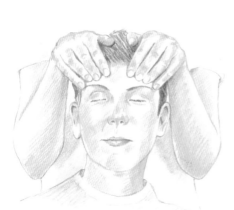

Step 7
Hook all four fingers gently under the cheekbones and hold this position for 3–5 seconds. Then do the same under the eyebrows.

Step 8
Now apply firm pressure into the skull with all four fingers on the forehead, just above the eyebrows. The techniques in steps 7 and 8 can help sinus conditions and lift "heavy" headaches.

Leave your partner to sit or lie quietly for a while. You may wish to use the clearing visualization, or break the energy connection between you (see page 31)

CHAPTER 10

SELF-MASSAGE

Self-massage is one of the best ways of learning how to be a good masseur – of discovering what feels good in the dual role of giver and receiver. It is an age-old form of healing and one we all turn to instinctively when we feel stiff or in pain – squeezing our tense shoulders or rubbing away a bruise. Many centuries ago, self-massage was used ritualistically by Mongolian warriors, to rid themselves of fear before going into battle. There are drawbacks to self-massage, however – mainly the difficulty of relaxing completely and of reaching all parts of the body without straining. But on the whole, any disadvantages are outweighed by the rewards. Nobody knows your body as well as you do, no-one but you can tell what feels best, nor locate so precisely where it hurts.

This chapter presents self-massage sequences that you can use at work, at home, or in the car, wherever you feel tense or tired, stiff or aching. The reflexology self-massage sequence works on the hands, where the reflexes are closer together than on the feet (see the charts on pages 248–9). Although this is less effective than a foot treatment, it is often more practical to work on the hands, as you can give yourself a discreet treatment wherever you are.

Before starting a self-massage treatment, familiarize yourself with the basic strokes, described in chapter 1. If you are treating yourself to a massage at home, create a healing, relaxing atmosphere by preparing yourself and the room following the guidelines on pages 28–30. For an aromatherapy massage, choose appropriate essential oils from the chart on page 250.

Wherever you are using self-massage, even at work, begin by sitting quietly for a few moments until your breathing begins to deepen. Then follow the centring meditation on page 30. You may also like to use the cleansing visualization (page 30) to create a healing space filled with protective energy.

At the end of the treatment, allow yourself time to rest. Then clear your energy and the energy of the space using the clearing visualization on page 31.

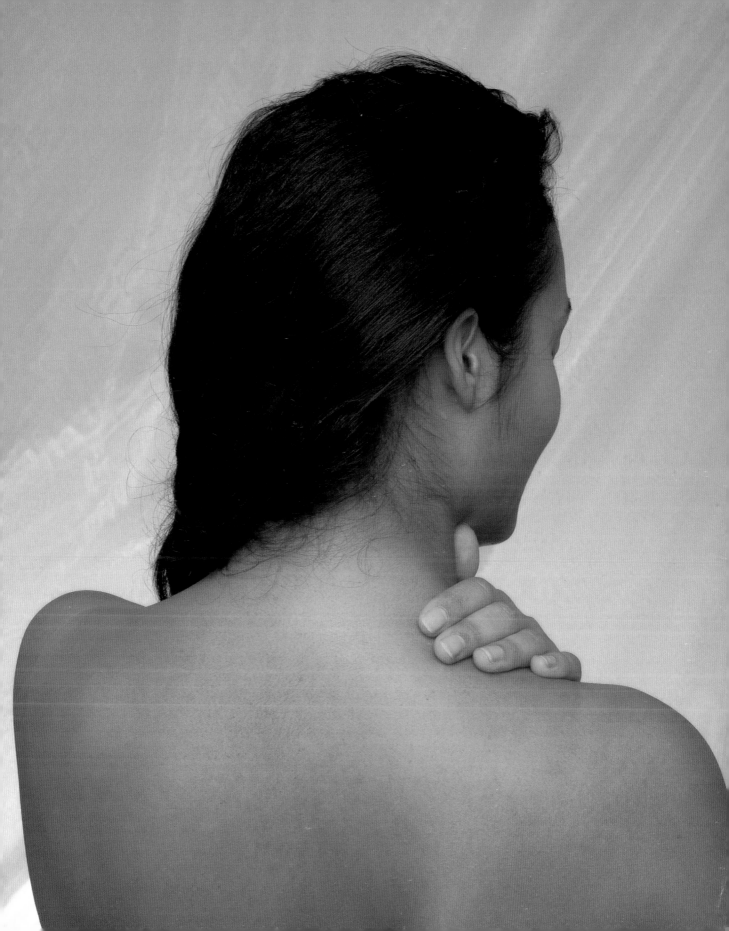

HOLISTIC SELF-MASSAGE

You can massage whichever parts of the body you can reach, using any of the strokes in the massage sequence described in chapter 2. But you will find it easiest to relax if you treat each part in the postions and order shown here, working from feet to head.

As you massage each part of your body in turn, start with a light caress and gradually work deeper, experimenting with different strokes and pressures. Allow enough time to acquaint yourself fully with each area of your body, so that you emerge feeling restored all over.

Caution: *See page 5 for a full list of cautions and contraindications for massage.*

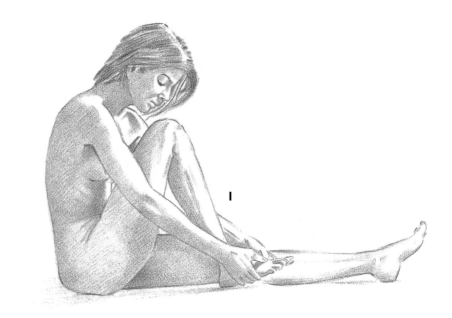

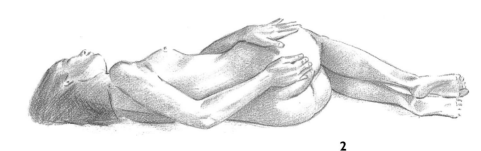

Step 1
Sit on the floor with your legs outstretched in front of you. Alternating between first the left side and then the right, work on your feet, ankles, lower legs, knee joints, and then your thighs from knee to hip.

Step 2
Lie on your back with your knees bent, feet on the floor. Massage your whole pelvic area, beginning with the inner triangle from the pubic bone, round between the legs to the sitting bone. Roll over onto one side to work on the area from sitting bone to coccyx, over the buttock, and round the pelvic bone and hip joint to the front. Roll over to your other side and repeat. Now massage your entire abdomen.

Step 3

Lying down, massage from your solar plexus to your collarbone. Pull along the sides of your chest, then work along between the ribs from the midline outward.

Step 4

Lying down, alternate between your two arms, starting with the left. First massage each hand, then each forearm including the elbow, and finally your upper arms to the armpits and shoulder joints.

Step 5

Lying down, press along the upper edge of your collarbone and the top of your shoulders. Massage the sides and back of your neck and as much of your shoulder blades and upper back as you can reach.

Step 6

Sitting down, work up from your pelvis as far as you can. Lying down on the floor, wriggle your back against a rolling pin or rubber ball; sitting, roll against a wall; standing, wriggle against the edge of a door.

Step 7

Lying down, stroke your whole face firmly from forehead to chin, working from the centre outward. Massage your jawbone and ears, then your whole scalp.

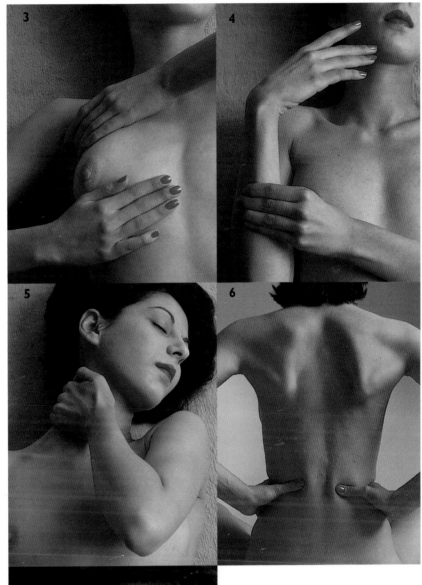

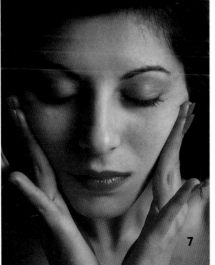

End by "connecting" your whole body by making long, sweeping, gliding strokes down your arms, down your body and down your legs to your feet. Lie quietly and rest.

CHINESE SELF-MASSAGE

This 15-minute self-care sequence promotes good general physical and emotional health.

For help in locating the acupoints to treat, consult the charts on pages 242–5.

Caution: *See page 5 for a full list of cautions and contraindications for massage.*

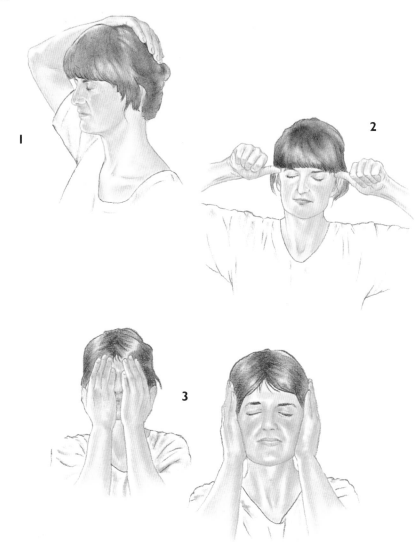

Step 1
Sitting comfortably on a chair or on the floor, place the heel of your right hand on the top of your head, midway between your ears, covering the acupoint Du20. Apply moderate pressure and knead the area slowly with circular strokes – 10 clockwise, then 10 anticlockwise. In Chinese medicine the brain is called the "Reservoir of Marrow", and Du20 controls the flow of Qi passing through it.

Caution: *Do not use firm pressure on the top of your head if you are elderly, or suffering from epilepsy, bone disease, or clinical depression.*

Step 2
Put your thumbs on the Taiyang points on your temples, one thumb width away from the outside edge of the eye and level with the top of the ear. Knead both points slowly in a clockwise direction and with moderate pressure, 30 times.

Step 3
Rub your hands together until they are warm. Then place your palms either side of your nose and slide them across your cheeks toward the ears with a smooth, wiping action. Repeat 10 times. This gentle massage increases the circulation of blood to the face and helps to prevent wrinkles.

Caution: *Do not perform this massage if you have acne or pimples.*

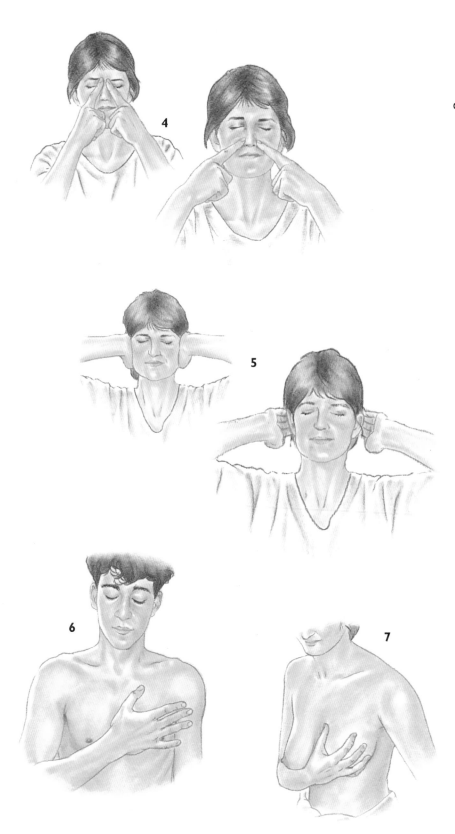

Step 4

Starting with your index fingers on either side of the bridge of your nose, push down along the sides of your nose toward the nostrils. Repeat 20 times, applying moderate pressure. This massage, "Pushing the Life Longer" in Chinese, stimulates several acupoints.

Step 5

Place your palms over your ears with your fingers pointing toward the back of your head. Press your palms down tightly and then remove them quickly. When you remove your palms, you may hear a sound like a drumbeat. Repeat 10 times. This exercise improves your hearing and prevents various ear diseases, particularly tinnitus.

Step 6

Rub your palms together to warm them. Then place the heel of your right hand on your breastbone, midway between the nipples, over Ren17. Apply moderate pressure and knead 40 clockwise circles, then 40 anticlockwise circles.

Step 7

With your right palm, rub around your left breast 20 times. Change hands and rub around your right breast 20 times. Then cup your left breast in your right hand, squeeze gently, and quickly release 20 times. Repeat the squeezing sequence on your right breast 20 times.

CHINESE SELF-MASSAGE

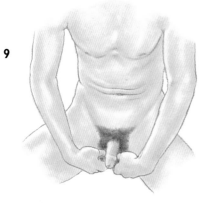

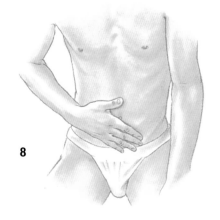

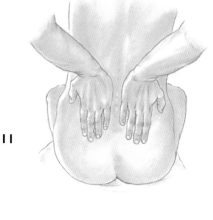

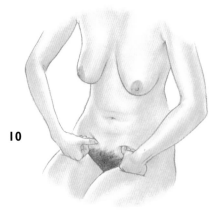

Step 8

Place your right palm on your abdomen and rub in a clockwise circle around the navel. Repeat 20 times, applying a little more pressure each time.

Then knead Ren4 with your right thumb, 50 to 100 times, alternating between clockwise and anticlockwise kneading. This massage is particularly beneficial when you are generally run down, or weak after illness, and it also aids digestion.

Caution: *Do not use steps 8, 10, and 11 if you are pregnant.*

Step 9 (for men only)

Hold your scrotum in your hands, squeeze gently, and then release. Repeat 50 times. If you prefer, you can do this massage through loose cotton underwear.

Step 10 (for women only)

With your thumbs, knead the St29 points, using moderate pressure. Make 50 small, circular kneading strokes.

Step 11

Place your hands on your lower back, on the B23 points either side of the spine. Rub the area with 50 to 100 fairly vigorous upward and downward strokes. Then slide your hands further down your back and repeat. This massage maintains the healthy functioning of the Kidneys (fundamental organs in Chinese medicine) and gives energy to the body.

Caution: *Do not massage the back region during menstruation.*

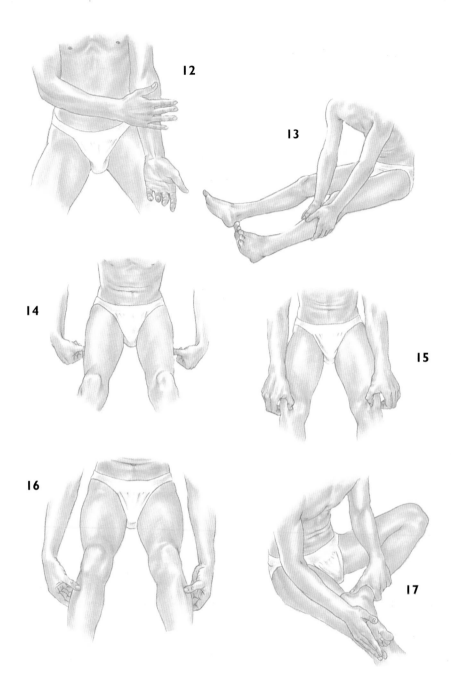

Step 12

Stretch your left arm in front of you, with your palm facing upward. With your right hand, rub your left arm from the wrist to just below the shoulder with a single, smooth, upward stroke. Turn your arm over so the palm is facing downward, then rub down it to complete one sequence. Repeat 20 times on the left arm, then 20 times on the right.

Step 13

Sit on the floor with your legs stretched out in front of you. Hold your left thigh with both hands and rub down the leg toward the ankle with some pressure, then up again, to complete one sequence. Repeat 20 times, then massage your right leg 20 times in the same way.

Step 14

Still sitting, press GB31 on each thigh 30 times with your thumbs.

Step 15

Find the two dimpled areas of each knee just below the kneecap. Knead these points in both knees 30 times, using your thumb and index finger and firm, circular strokes.

Step 16

Press acupoint St36 on each leg 30 times, with your thumbs. St36 is one of the energy-giving acupoints.

Caution: *Do not massage St36 if you are pregnant.*

Step 17

Bend your left leg and rest your left foot on your right thigh. Rub your palms together until they are warm, then place your right palm on the sole of your left foot. Rub up and down over the area 30 times. Repeat on your right foot.

To finish, use gentle, sweeping strokes up to your knees and down to your feet, three times. On the third sweep, continue up your legs to your hips and then down to your knees three times. Then sweep up your body to your shoulders and back down to your hips three times. Sit or lie quietly and rest for a while.

REIKI SELF-TREATMENT

This complete sequence will take about 45 minutes. It will leave you feeling relaxed, reduce stress, and strengthen resistance to illness.

Sit or lie down, as you feel most comfortable. Lay your hands gently on the different body positions and remain in each position for 3–5 minutes. If you have pains or definite problem areas, let your hands rest there for 10–20 minutes. Simply be creative with your hands – let yourself be led by them and follow your intuition.

Step 1

Place your hands over your eyes, resting your palms on the cheekbones. This position helps colds, produces clarity of thought, helps stress reduction and intuition, and facilitates meditation.

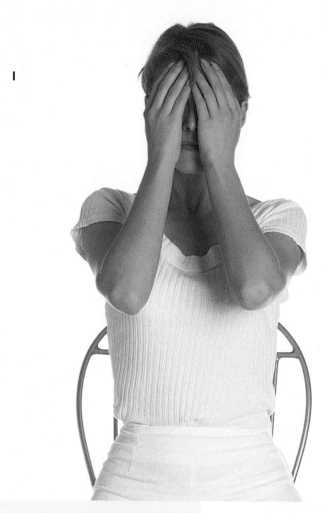

Step 2

Place your hands on both sides of your head, above your ears, touching your temples. This position harmonizes the two sides of the brain, improves memory and enjoyment of life, and is helpful for depression and headaches.

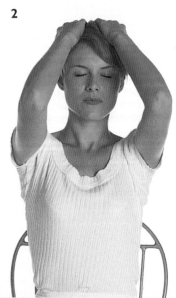

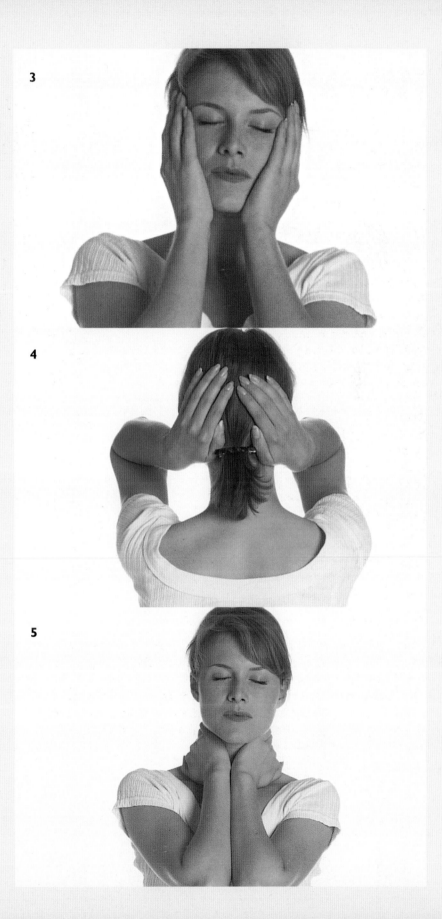

Step 3

Place your hands on both sides of your head, covering your ears. This position is very comforting and affects the whole body. It is helpful for earache and eases the symptoms of colds and flu.

Step 4

Place your hands on the back of your head, holding your head like a ball. This position eases sleep disorders, conveys a sense of security, promotes intuition, helps headaches, relieves fears and depression, and calms the mind and the emotions.

Step 5

Place your hands around your throat, wrists touching in the centre. This position harmonizes blood pressure and metabolism, helps neck pain and hoarseness, and promotes self-expression.

REIKI SELF-TREATMENT

Step 6

Place your hands on the left and right sides of your upper chest, fingers touching just below the collarbone. This position strengthens the immune system, regulates heart and blood pressure, stimulates lymph circulation, increases the capacity for love and enjoyment of life, and transforms negativity.

Step 7

Place your hands over your lower ribcage above the waist, fingers touching. This position regulates the digestion, gives energy, promotes relaxation, and reduces fears and frustrations.

Step 8

Place your hands on either side of your navel, fingers touching. This position regulates sugar and fat metabolism and digestion, and helps ease powerful emotions such as fear, depression, and frustration. It can also help to increase self-confidence.

Step 9

Place your hands over your pubic bone, in the shape of a "V". For women, the fingertips should touch. This position treats the large intestine, bladder, urethra, and sexual organs, eases menstrual disorders in women, provides grounding, and helps existential fear.

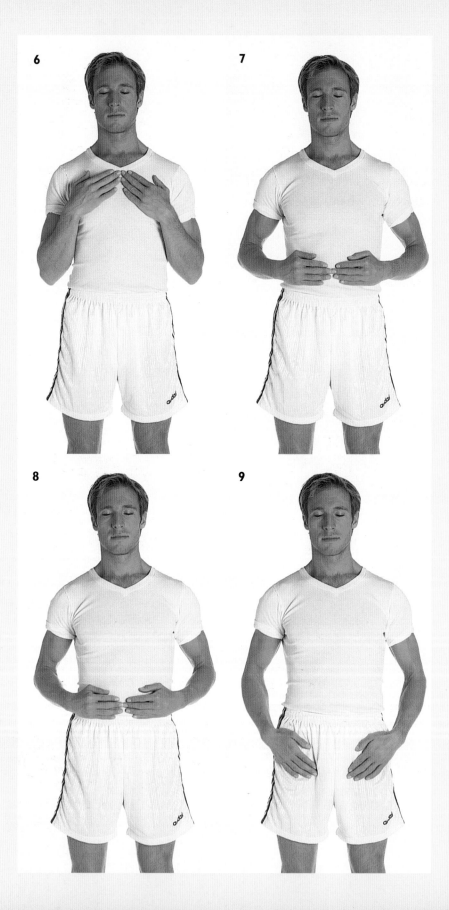

Step 10

Place your hands on your upper shoulders, on either side of your spine. This position is helpful for shoulder tension, back, and neck problems, promotes relaxation, releases blocked emotions, and helps problems with responsibility.

Step 11

Place one hand in the middle of your chest and the other at the same height on your back. This position balances the thymus gland, harmonizes the heart, stimulates the immune system, and increases enjoyment of life and confidence. It also helps worries and depression.

Step 12

Place your hands around your waist at kidney height, fingers pointing toward your spine. This position strengthens the kidneys, adrenal glands, and nerves, promotes detoxification, relaxes stress, eases back pains, and reinforces self-esteem and confidence.

Step 13

Place your hands so that your fingers touch your coccyx, your hands opening into a "V". This position treats the sexual organs, digestion, and the sciatic nerve, promotes creativity and confidence, and provides grounding.

Finish this sequence with the clearing visualization on page 31. Rest quietly for a while.

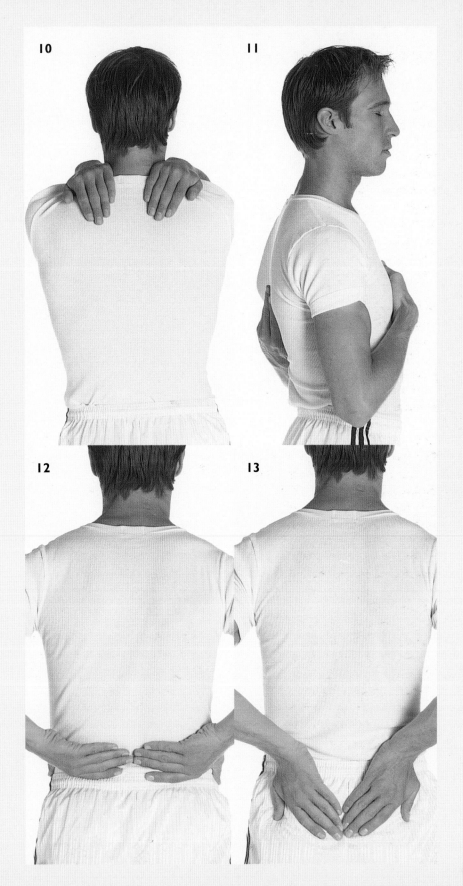

AROMATHERAPY SELF-MASSAGE

Choose your essential oils carefully, referring to the chart on page 250. Prepare your massage oil following the guidelines on pages 28–9.

Caution: *See page 5 for a full list of cautions and contraindications for massage.*

Step 1

Place the pads of the middle three fingers of each hand on your brow between your eyes. Using light pressure, move your hands apart across the brow to the corners of each eye. Apply gentle, circular pressure around the hollows on the outside of each eye bone. Use your 4th finger only to stroke under the eyes back toward the nose.

Return to the forehead and repeat the movement.

Step 2

With your fingers pointing up and your thumbs underneath your jawbone, press along the top of your cheekbones. Start either side of your nose and work out to your temples, then return lightly to the centre. Work outward again along the middle of the cheekbones.

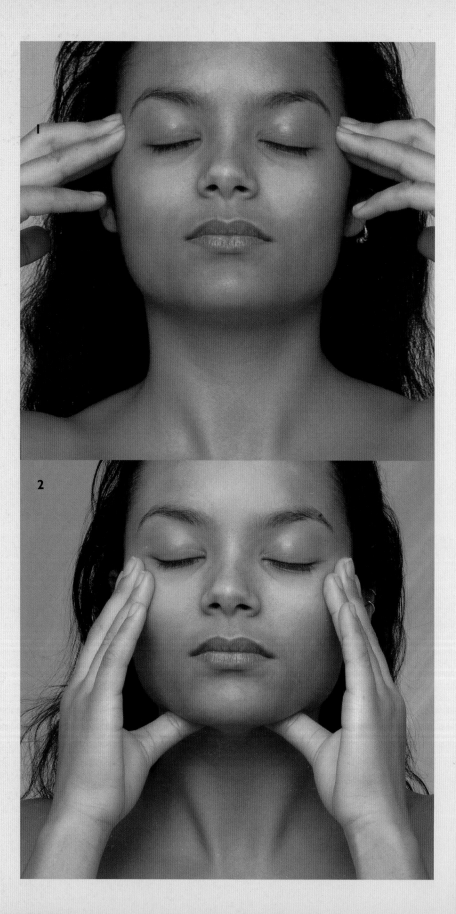

Step 3

Place your whole hand gently over the opposite shoulder, with your palm resting on the collarbone and your fingers resting on the shoulder muscle. Move your hand firmly along the top of your shoulder to your neck. Continue up your neck as far as you can and then massage behind the ears. Return lightly to the shoulder. Repeat several times.

Caution: *Do not massage the midpoint of the top of the shoulder if you are pregnant.*

Step 4

Feel with your fingers for knotty, painful areas in your shoulder muscle. Apply firm, circular pressure to any tension nodules you find, using the pads of your fingers. Finish by repeating step 3.

Repeat steps 3 and 4 on the other shoulder.

Step 5

Gently grip the top of your left wrist with your right hand. Apply firm pressure and slide your hand up to the shoulder. Use a light stroke to return to the wrist. Repeat several times.

Step 6

Applying pressure with the pad of your thumb, make wide circles around the area on the inside of your wrist. Then repeat step 5, this time sliding your hand up the inside of your arm. On the last stroke, pull off firmly and slowly over the hand.

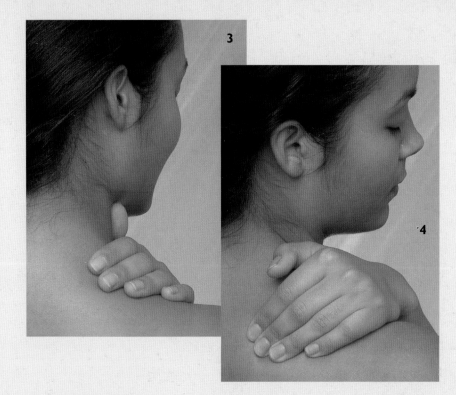

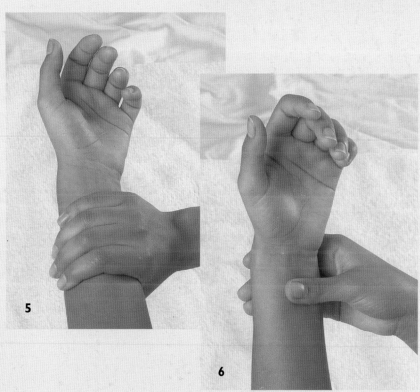

Repeat steps 5 and 6 on the other arm.

AROMATHERAPY
SELF-MASSAGE

Step 7
Place your palm flat on your chest and, using firm pressure, make large clockwise circles. Using your finger pads to apply pressure, continue up the neck and behind your ears.

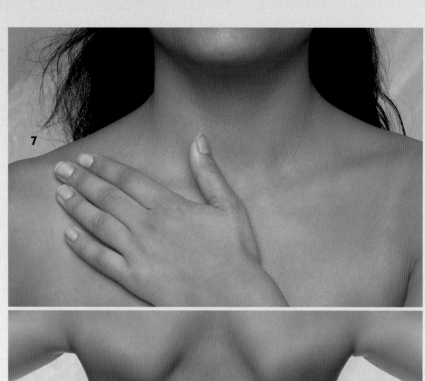

Step 8
Place your hands under your ribcage, with your thumbs at the front of your waist. Using your finger pads, massage in small circles over the muscle tissue to either side of your spine. Work out toward the sides of the body.

Step 9
Lie down on your back and place the palm of one hand on your solar plexus, the soft area directly beneath the breastbone. With the palm of your other hand, massage gently in a large clockwise circle round your navel. Start at the right side of the pubic bone and work up that side of the abdomen. Continue across the stomach just below the other hand, and on down the other side of the abdomen, back to your starting point.

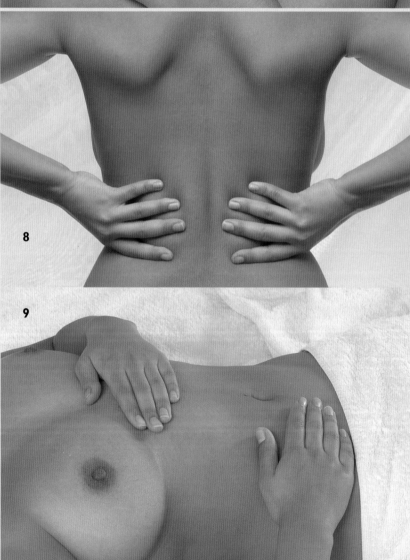

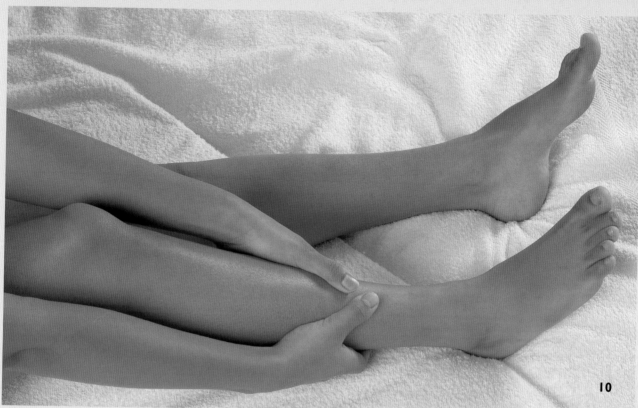

10

Step 10

Return to sitting and place the fingers of both hands on the underside of your right ankle, with the thumbs on the top. Stroke firmly up the leg to the knee, then use a light stroke to return to the foot. Continue with the same movement from your knee to the top of your thigh, using a light return stroke.

Caution: *Take care not to apply pressure in a downward direction on your legs, since this is not helpful to the circulation.*

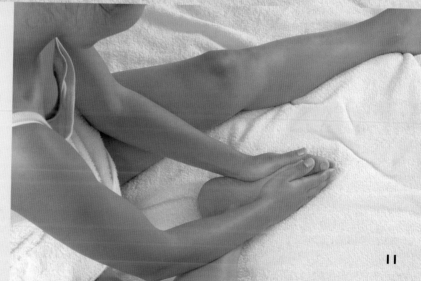

11

Step 11

Take your right foot between your hands so that the palm of your left hand rests in the arch. Pressing firmly, slowly draw your hands down to the tip of the foot in a "sandwich" stroke.

Repeat steps 10 and 11 on the left leg.

Lie or sit comfortably and cover yourself with a towel to keep warm. You may wish to use the clearing visualization on page 31. Relax for 5–10 minutes.

REFLEXOLOGY SELF-TREATMENT

For the maximum possible benefit, reflexology is always applied to "the very roots of our being" – the feet. However, for self-treatment, you can use reflexology on your hands.

For help in locating the reflexes, see the hand maps on pages 248–9.

Caution: *See page 5 for a full list of cautions and contraindications for massage.*

Follow the complete sequence of exercises on the right hand before treating the left hand.

I

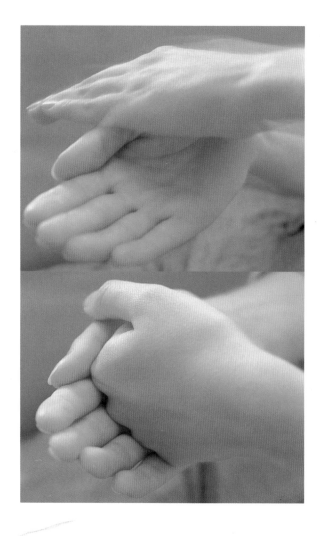

Step 1
Warm up your hand by rubbing the outside edge of your thumb with your other palm. Then knead your palm with the fist of your other hand.

Step 2
Creep your thumb along the diaphragm line.

2

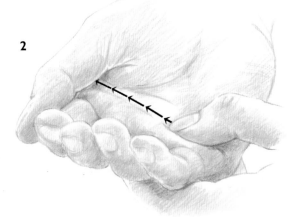

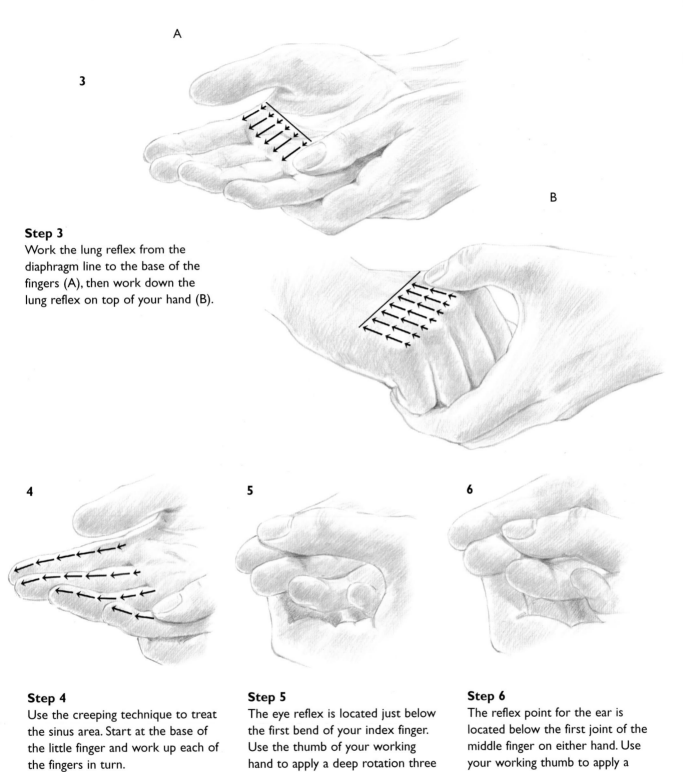

A

3

B

Step 3
Work the lung reflex from the diaphragm line to the base of the fingers (A), then work down the lung reflex on top of your hand (B).

4

5

6

Step 4
Use the creeping technique to treat the sinus area. Start at the base of the little finger and work up each of the fingers in turn.

Step 5
The eye reflex is located just below the first bend of your index finger. Use the thumb of your working hand to apply a deep rotation three or four times.

Step 6
The reflex point for the ear is located below the first joint of the middle finger on either hand. Use your working thumb to apply a deep rotation three or four times.

Step 7

Work all around the base of the thumb, using the creeping technique, to treat the neck and thyroid areas.

Step 8

The coccyx reflex lies at the base of the spinal reflex, along the edge of the base of the thumb. Apply firm pressure with the four fingers of your working hand.

Step 9

The hip, pelvis, and sciatic reflex points are located on top of the hands below the little finger. To contact this area, apply pressure with your four working fingers to the outside edge of the hand you are treating.

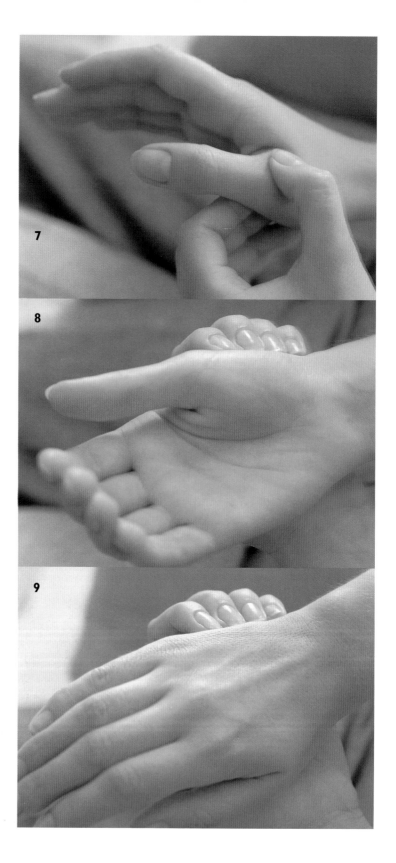

Step 10
Creep along the entire spinal reflex from the base of the hand and up the outside edge of the thumb.

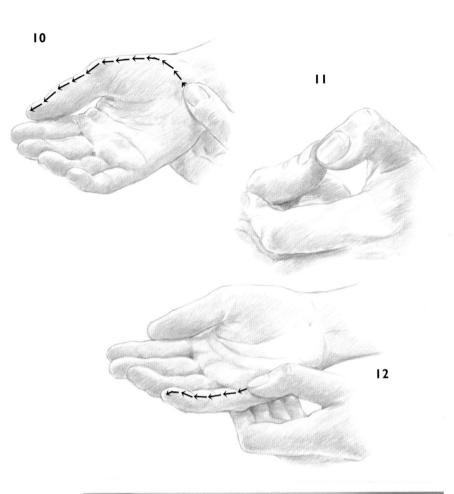

Step 11
Apply firm pressure to the top of your thumb with your working thumb, to stimulate the brain.

Step 12
Use your thumb to creep up the shoulder reflex on the little finger, from the diaphragm line. This reflex overlaps the sinus area.

Step 13
The small, triangular reflex point for the knee and elbow is on top of the hand, below the little finger. It sits between the diaphragm and waist lines. Creep across this area with your working fingers.

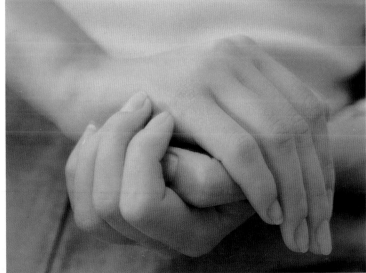

Step 14

Creep your thumb across the palm of your left hand only, to contact the stomach, pancreas, and spleen.

Step 15

Creep across your palm in parallel lines, as shown. On the right hand you will work the liver, gall bladder, ileocecal valve, and ascending and transverse colon, while on the left hand you will contact reflex points for the transverse, descending, and sigmoid colon.

Step 16

To contact reflexes for the bladder, work up the fleshy part of the thumb using the creeping technique. Continue up the hand toward the base of your index finger, which will also work the ureter tube.

The kidney reflex is above the ureter tube. Carry on working up the fleshy part of the thumb until you reach the diaphragm line. Apply a deep rotation to this area to work the kidney.

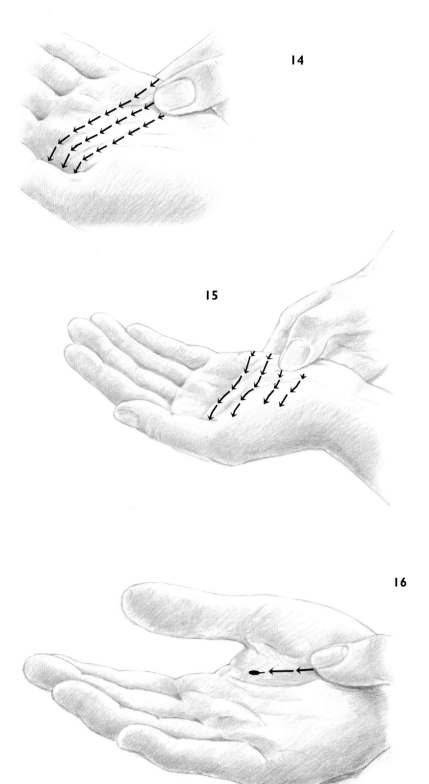

Caution: *Do not use steps 17 to 19 if you are pregnant.*

Step 17
Find the uterus/prostate reflex on the edge of your wrist, below the thumb. Apply pressure to this area with the middle finger of your working hand.

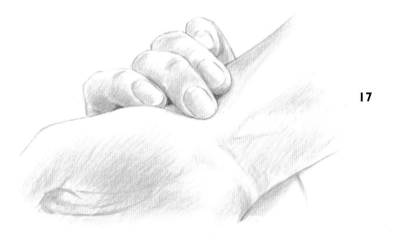

17

Step 18
Use your middle finger to work the ovary/testis reflex on the edge of the hand, below the little finger and in front of the wrist bone.

18

Step 19
Continue all the way around your wrist to contact the fallopian tube/vas deferens reflex, using all four fingers of your working hand.

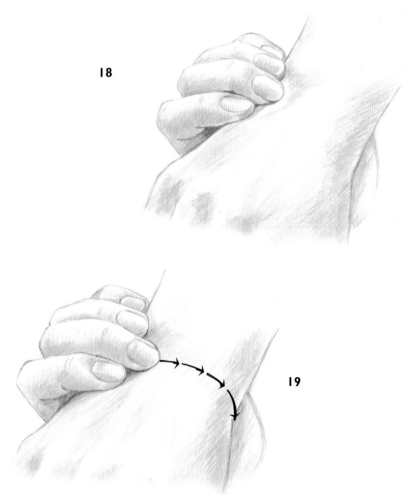

Sit quietly and rest for a while. You may wish to use the clearing visualization on page 31.

19

HEAD SELF-MASSAGE

This 20-minute self-care routine is designed to relax, re-energize, tone, and release your head, neck, and shoulders, and to stimulate energy throughout your whole body.

Caution: *If you have a history of neck problems, consult your doctor before using steps 1 to 4.*

See page 5 for a full list of cautions and contraindications for massage.

Step 1

Clench the fist of one hand and beat with your knuckles on the opposite side of your neck. Work a line down from the base of your skull to the outside edge of your shoulder. Do this as hard as you can bear, two or three times, then change hands and repeat on the other side.

Caution: *Do not massage the midpoint of the top of the shoulder if you are pregnant.*

Step 2

Starting again at the base of your skull, knead with your fingers down the opposite side of your neck and across your shoulders, along the same line as in step 1. Press as hard as you can. Then change hands and repeat on the other side.

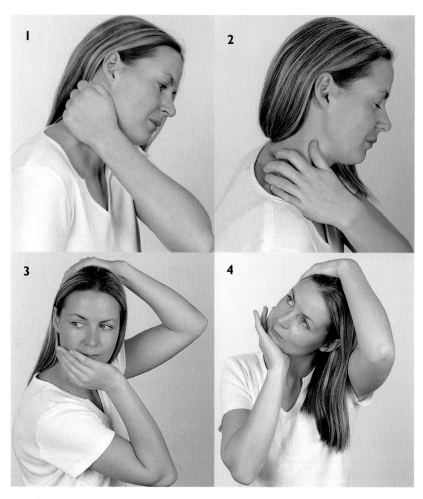

Step 3

Hold the top right side of your head with your left hand, and place the heel of your right hand on the left side of your chin. Pulling with your left hand and pushing with your right, gently twist your head round to the right as far as you can. Hold this position for a count of 30, then slowly release and bring your head back to centre. Change hands and repeat on the other side, this time turning to the left.

Step 4

Still holding your head as in step 3, push with your right hand and pull with your left, gently tilting your head over to the left, with your ear moving toward your shoulder. Hold for a count of 30, then release slowly and bring your head back upright. Change hands and repeat, this time tilting your head to the right. If you cannot maintain the hold for a count of 30, start with a count of 10 and build up slowly.

Step 5

Scratch vigorously all over your head to loosen up your scalp. Then comb your fingers through your hair to remove any knots.

Step 6

With your fingers apart, push your hands up into your hair, close to the scalp. Bring your fingers together to grip the hair and pull them out along its length. Hold for 3–5 seconds, then release. Repeat this pulling, moving your hands slightly each time, until you have covered your whole head.

Step 7

Place the pads of the fingers of one hand along the midline on the top of your head, with the little finger on the hairline and the others roughly 1 cm (0.5 in) apart. Rotate your fingers with firm pressure for 3–5 seconds. Move two finger widths back along the midline and repeat, continuing until you reach the base of the skull.

Now start again at the hairline and work lines two finger widths either side of the midline, using both hands at the same time. Continue in this way, finishing with a line just above the ears. Then rub vigorously all over your head.

Caution: *Do not use firm pressure on the top of your head if you are elderly, or suffering from epilepsy, bone disease, or clinical depression.*

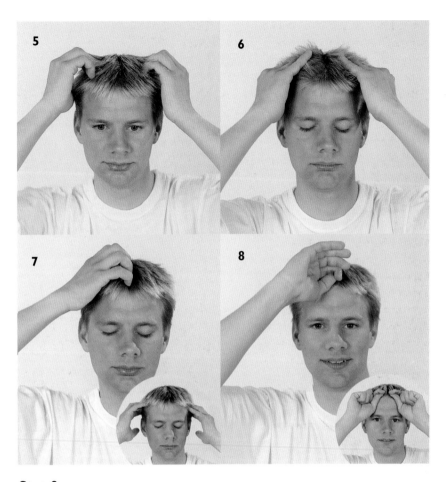

Step 8

Take a small section of hair at the centre of the hairline and pull gently for 3–5 seconds. If your hair is long enough, wrap a small twist around your finger to ensure an even tension. Release, move two finger widths back along the midline and repeat. Continue until you reach the nape of the neck.

Return to the hairline and, using both hands, work two parallel lines two finger widths from the midline. When you reach the neck, run your fingers back up through the hair to ease out your scalp. Then work two more parallel lines back from the hairline. Repeat until you have covered your whole head.

HEAD SELF-MASSAGE

Step 9

Comb your fingers through your hair to loosen it. Place the fingertips of one hand along the midline on the top of the head, with your little finger on the hairline and fingers about 1 cm (0.5 in) apart. Press evenly and firmly for 3–5 seconds. Release and repeat, moving four finger widths back each time, until you reach the nape of the neck.

Now start again at the hairline and work back across the head in parallel lines two finger widths from the first line, using both hands simultaneously. Try to work smoothly and rhythmically. Continue working parallel lines at two finger width intervals until you reach your ears. Feel the tension draining away.

Step 10

This time start at the base of the neck, with the fingers of both hands either side of the spine. Press as hard as you can into your neck and hold for about 5 seconds, then release. Move four finger widths up toward the crown and repeat, moving up the neck and over the top of your head to the hairline.

Now return to the base of the neck and work two parallel lines two finger widths from the first. Repeat in this way until you have covered your whole head. Feel the tension lifting from your head.

Caution: *Do not apply strong pressure directly on your spine.*

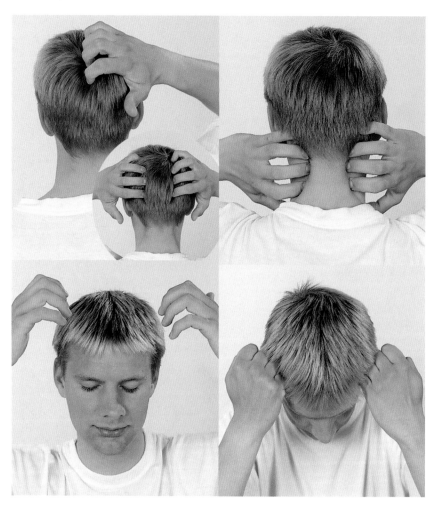

Step 11

Tap all over your head with the fingertips of both hands. Your hands should bounce off your hair lightly and rhythmically.

Step 12

Loosely clench your fists and use knuckling to work firmly over your head. Starting at the base of the skull, work from side to side across the back of the head in parallel lines, moving up two finger widths each time. Then move to above your ears and do the same on the sides of your head. Finish with a firm knuckling over the top. Scratch your head vigorously all over.

Steps 13 to 18 exercise and massage your eye muscles.

Step 13

Hold your hands about 20 cm (8 in) in front of your face, with the palms facing each other 7 cm (3 in) apart. Be aware of the space between your hands and allow yourself to feel the flow of energy between your palms. Turn your palms to face you, slowly moving them closer to you, until you can sense the energy flowing ino your eyes. Spend a moment or two with your eyes closed, feeling the strength of the energy flowing into them.

Step 14

Still with your eyes closed, tense and relax the muscles within your eyes rhythmically for a count of 20. Then open your eyes and move your hands away from your face, holding one hand at full arm's length, the other about half way. Focus on one hand and then the other, moving your gaze quickly between them, for a count of 20.

Step 15

Place your palms lightly over your eyes, taking care not to press on the lids. Feel the heat and energy from your palms relaxing your eyes. Tense and relax the muscles for a count of 20.

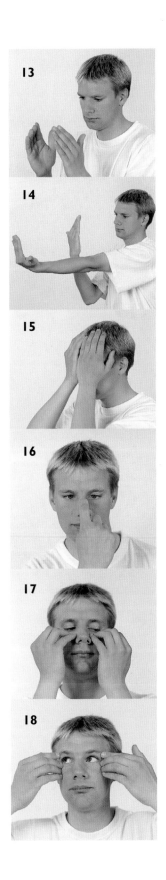

Step 16

With one finger, massage the bridge of your nose with small circular movements for 2–3 seconds. Look at your finger as you massage, crossing your eyes. Work down the length of the nose and back up again, following your finger with your eyes. Repeat twice more, then repeat step 15.

Step 17

Place the tips of the four fingers of each hand in a line under your eyebrows and rotate gently. As you do so, move your eyes along from the tip of one index finger, along the other tips, to the other index finger, and back again. Repeat this slowly five times. Now move your fingers to underneath your eyes, just above the line of the cheekbone. Massage gently with rotations and move your eyes along the line of your fingertips, repeating five times, as before. Rest and relax your eyes by repeating step 15.

Step 18

Place the tips of the four fingers of each hand beside the outer edge of the eyes, in a vertical line. Rotate them gently as you move your eyes down from the index to the little finger of one hand, and then the other. Repeat this slowly, five times. Finally, relax your eyes by repeating step 15 again.

HEAD SELF-MASSAGE

Caution: *Do not massage the sides of the face, the throat, across the chin, or behind the ears if you have cancer. Do not massage your throat if you are pregnant.*

Step 19
Start at the base of your throat, with your three middle fingers in a horizontal line either side of your larynx. Rotate your fingers firmly for 3–5 seconds, then move up two finger widths and repeat. Continue up your throat and under your chin.

Step 20
Use your thumbs to make rotations with firm pressure under the jawbone, starting by the base of the ears. Rotate in one position for 3–5 seconds, then move two finger widths along the jawbone and repeat, until your thumbs meet in the middle under your chin.

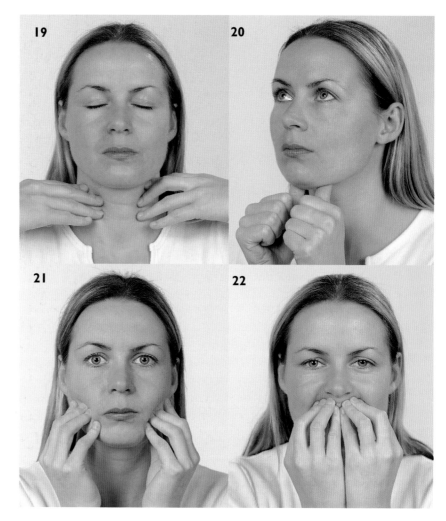

Step 21
Next knead firmly along your bottom gums, using the four fingers of each hand. Start in front of your ears, massaging firmly down into the gum for 3–5 seconds and then moving two finger widths along the gum line to repeat. Continue until your hands meet on your chin.

Step 22
Starting in front of your ears, knead along your top gum as in step 21, this time massaging up over the gum. Your hands should meet just under your nose.

Step 23

Starting in front of the ears again, and using both hands simultaneously, use all four fingers to make light rotations along the cheekbones. Rotate for 3–5 seconds in each position, moving two finger widths along each time. Be very gentle under the eyes.

Step 24

Use the three middle fingers of both hands to rotate firmly in the hollow of your temples for 3–5 seconds.

Step 25

Hold the four fingers of each hand so the tips are level and use them to tap firmly all over your face and throat. Work rhythmically with both hands together, wrists loose so the fingers bounce off your skin.

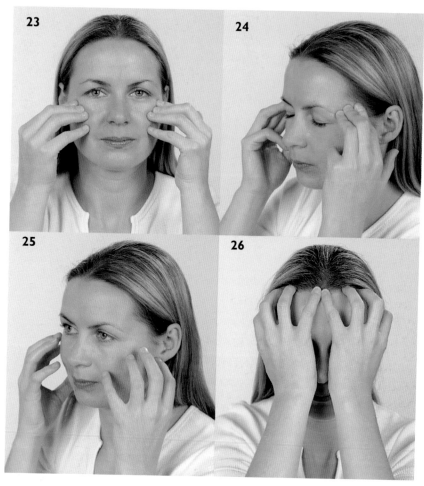

Step 26

Place the four fingers of each hand on your forehead, in a horizontal line just below the hairline. Feel the muscles in your forehead beneath your fingers, and tense and release these 10 times. The movement is tiny: keep your eyebrows still. Move your fingers two finger widths down your face, tensing and releasing the muscles under your fingertips, until you have covered your whole face and throat.

With practice you will become more aware of these muscles and find it easier to tense them.

Gently rest your hands side by side on the top of your head with your elbows together in front of your face. Close your eyes and spend a few moments on the clearing visualization on page 31, which will help to clear your aura, leaving you energized and refreshed.

CHAPTER 11

MASSAGE FOR RELAXATION

Relaxation is simply a transformation of your energy. Normally your energy is motivated: moving toward a goal somewhere else. Somehow you have to achieve your goal; later you will relax. This kind of energy can dominate your life, continually changing into something else that you have to achieve. The goal is always on the horizon. You go on running, but the distance to the goal remains the same.

However, there is another dimension to energy – unmotivated energy. The goal is in the present, here and now. When the goal is not in the future there is nothing to be achieved. This moment is relaxation. And in this moment an overflow of energy, a response, or an unprepared action is taking place. You can do things and still remain relaxed. But how can you reach this state?

Relaxation starts with the body – if you can relax your body, you will soon be able to relax your mind too. Loving touch can be a wonderful relaxant. Simply getting someone who cares for you to hold you close is an excellent way of relieving stress.

This chapter gives step-by-step instructions for effective relaxation techniques using holistic massage, aromatherapy, Chinese massage, and Reiki. These can either be used on their own, or incorporated into other massage treatments. Before giving the massage, prepare yourself and the room following the guidelines on pages 28–30. Begin by centring yourself, and if you wish, use the cleansing visualization and make the energy connection between you (pages 30–31).

The following sections of the massage sequences in chapters 2 to 10 are also particularly effective for relaxation and stress relief.

Caution: *See page 5 for a full list of cautions and contraindications for massage.*

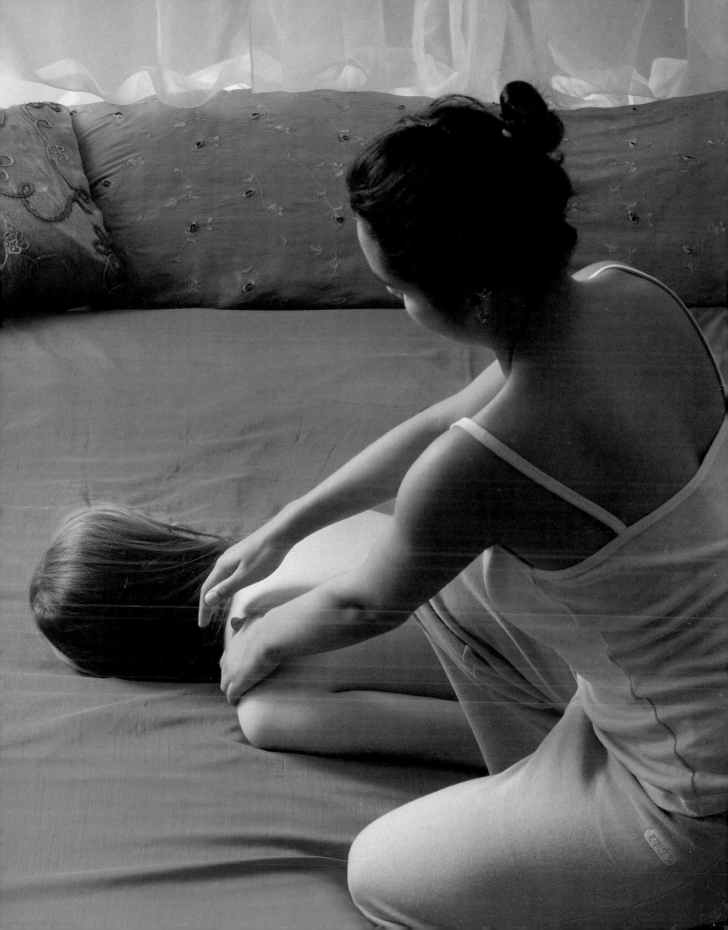

SINGLE STROKE FULL-BODY TREATMENT

This massage uses the Tiger's Claw stroke over the whole body, working with both hands at the same time. The light touch melts away tension in the muscles and encourages deeper breathing. The direction of the strokes follows the rising Yang and descending Yin energy, promoting smooth energy flow in the Channels (see page 15).

Step 1

Ask your partner to lie on her front. Hold your hands in a claw shape with strong fingers. Starting at the ankles, lightly stroke up the backs of the calves to the knees – the hands are strong but the touch is light. Then move your hands to the outsides of the legs and stroke back down to the feet. Repeat three times, ending on the up-stroke, just behind the knees.

Step 2

Starting at the knees, continue the upward stroke up the backs of the legs and over the buttocks to the hips. Move your hands to the outside of the body and stroke downward to the knees. Repeat three times, ending on the up-stroke, level with the hips.

Step 3

Now continue the up-stroke to the shoulders, with your hands either side of the spine. Move your hands out to the arms and stroke down the inner arms to the hands. Stroke up the outside of the arms and down the inside three times, ending on an up-stroke at the shoulders.

Step 4

Stroke both hands down your partner's sides to the hips. Move in toward the spine and stroke upward toward the shoulders. Repeat this three times, ending at the neck.

Step 5

To work on the neck and head, use only the thumb and first two fingers in a "claw" shape. Lightly stroke up the centre back of the neck to the crown of the head. Move your fingers out to each side of the head and stroke down to the base of the neck. Repeat three times.

Step 6

Ask your partner to turn over. Starting at the head, using only the thumb and first two fingers in your "claw", lightly stroke down the centre of the face and throat. At the base of the neck, move your hands out to the sides and stroke up over the ears to the top of the head. Repeat three times, ending at the base of the neck on a down-stroke.

Step 7

For the rest of the sequence, use all your fingers in your "claw" hands. Move out to the arms and continue the down-stroke over the outer sides of the arms, ending at the hands. Stroke up the inner arms to the shoulders. Repeat three times, ending on an up-stroke at the shoulders.

Step 8

Move your hands back to the sternum (top of the chest). With one hand following the other, stroke down the midline of the body to the Hara (lower abdomen). From here, move your hands out to your partner's sides and stroke upward. Repeat three times, ending on a sideways stroke, stopping level with the tops of the thighs.

Step 9

Stroke down the fronts of the legs to the knees. Move your hands to the outsides of the legs and stroke upward to the tops of the thighs. Repeat three times, ending on a down-stroke at the knees.

Step 10

Continue the down-stroke to the feet. Do not work on the soles, as a light touch will tickle, destroying the relaxing effect. Move your hands to the outsides of the ankles and stroke up the legs to the knees. Repeat three times, ending at the feet. Hold the feet for a few moments to end the massage.

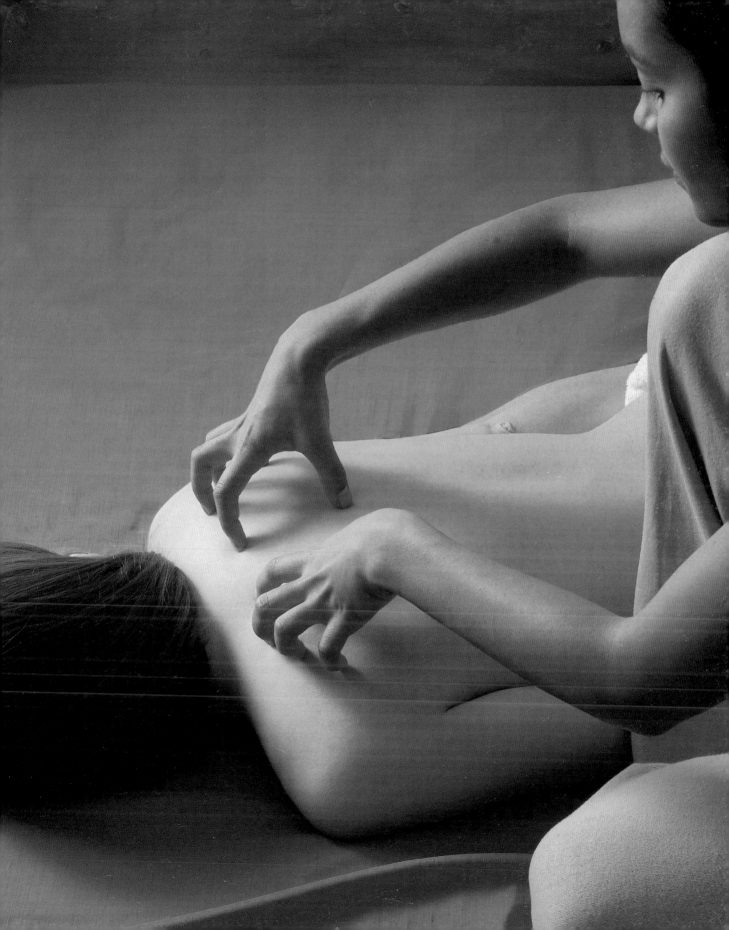

AROMATHERAPY MASSAGE FOR RELAXATION

The Relaxing Blend mixture of essential oils decribed below promotes relaxation. Use it for the whole-body massage described in chapter 7 (pages 154–69), or for self-massage on the shoulders (pages 208–11).

RELAXING BLEND

15 ml (2.5 tsp) carrier oil

2 drops Geranium

2 drops Lavender

2 drops Sandalwood

1 drop Ylang Ylang

Add the essential oils to the carrier oil in a screw-top bottle, replace the lid, and shake well. Warm the oil before use, by standing the bottle in a bowl of hot water.

For suggestions for suitable carrier oils, see page 29.

Caution: *Do not use Lavender oil in early pregnancy if there is a history of miscarriage.*

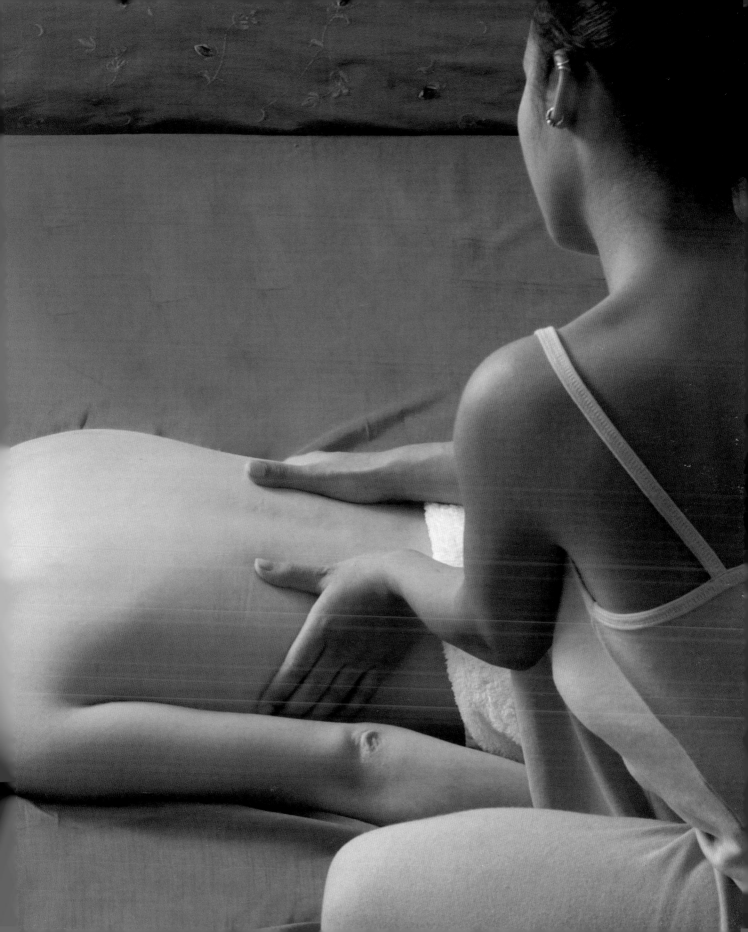

CHINESE MASSAGE FOR STRESS RELIEF

Chinese medicine views tension as the result of blocked Qi. This treatment smooths the flow of Qi and transforms tension from the upper body into vital energy. Follow the steps described to treat a partner or yourself.

For more help in locating the points to treat, see pages 242–5.

Step 1

With your thumb, apply pressure in small circles to the Liv3 points on both feet, in the furrow on the top of the foot between the 1st and 2nd toes, where the bones merge.

Step 2

Use your thumbs to apply circular pressure to the LI4 points on both hands, in the web between the thumb and index finger on the back of the hand.

Caution: *Do not massage this point on anyone who is pregnant.*

Step 3

Use both thumbs to apply circular pressure to point Du20 in the middle of the top of the head, between the ears.

Caution: *Do not massage this point on anyone who has high blood pressure.*

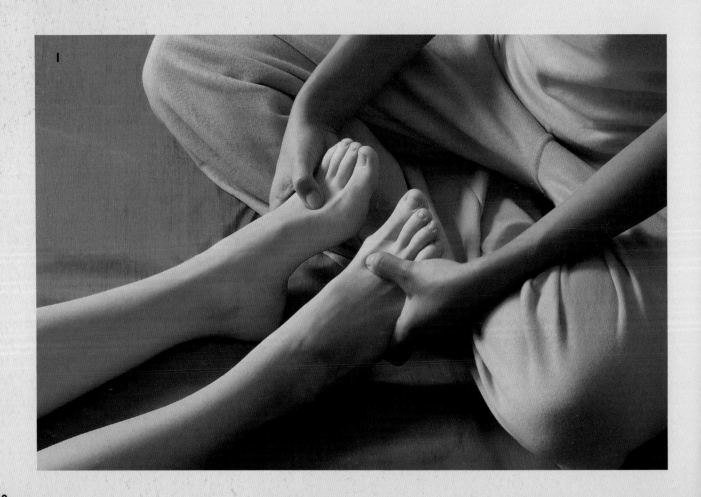

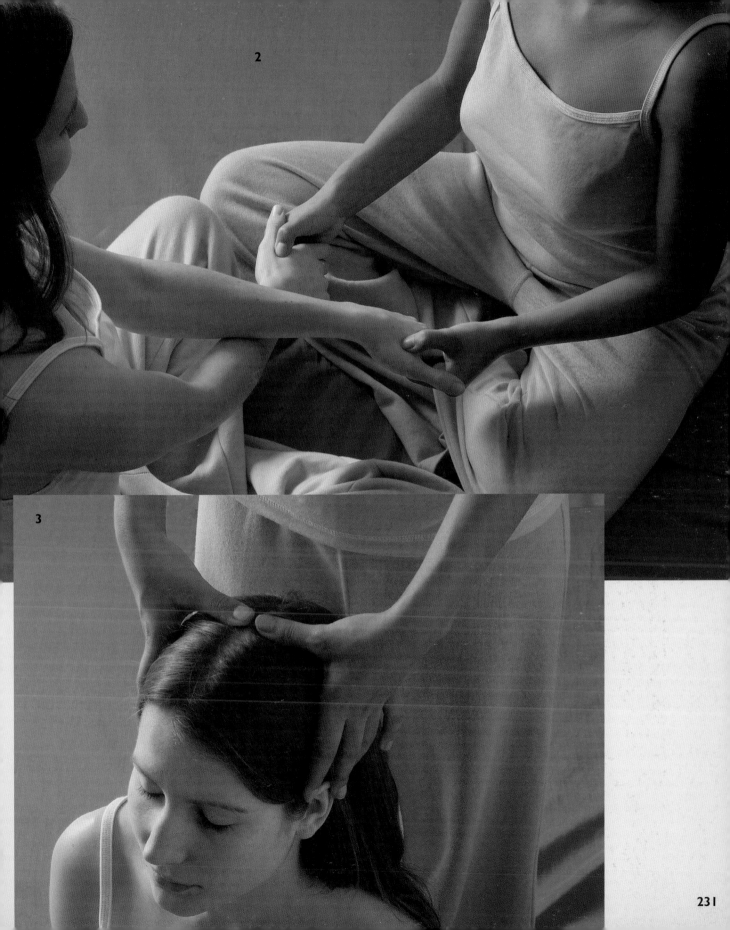

REIKI RELAXATION TECHNIQUE

Talk to your body

This exercise will help you to get in touch with your body more easily and consciously release any tension. You acknowledge your body as a friend and understand it better. Do this exercise once or twice a day, for 5–10 minutes or longer.

Step 1

Lie down or sit in a relaxed position. Then close your eyes. Now go with your consciousness inside your body. Look for any tension in your body, from your toes to your head.

Step 2

If you feel any tension anywhere, talk to that part of your body as if you were talking to a friend. Build up a dialogue between yourself and your body. Ask some questions: "How are you?" "Can I do anything for you?" "Can I release any tension or pain for you?" Then wait for an answer.

Step 3

Thank your body for being so helpful and "there" for you, functioning endlessly and keeping you going.

Step 4

Tell your body to relax and that there is nothing to fear. Tell it that you are there to take care of it. Slowly you will learn how to do this. Then your body will become fully relaxed.

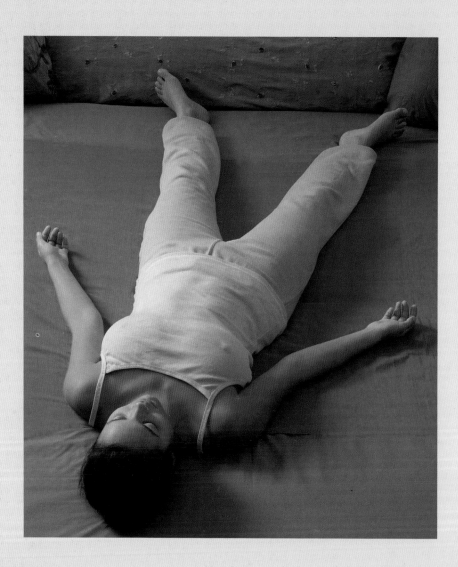

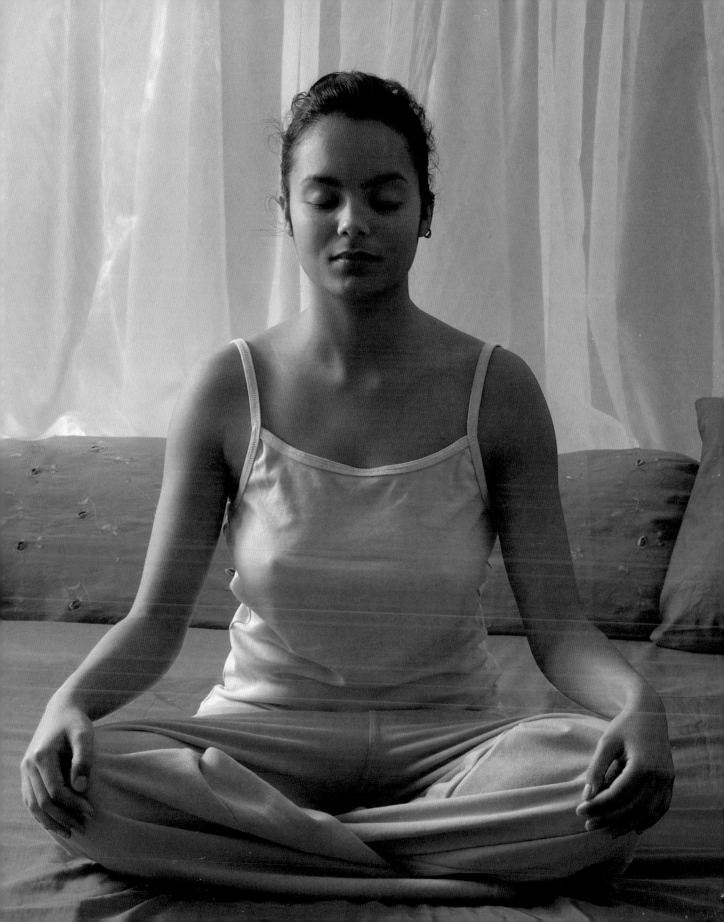

CHAPTER 12

TANTRIC SEXUAL MASSAGE

Tantra arose deep in Indian pre-history, from the merging of two distinct religious approaches. One claimed the supreme origin of life to be female (Shakti), the other masculine (Shiva). Tantric sages understood that the essence of life is in the meeting of opposite yet complementary polarities. From their belief that everything existing in the heavens and on earth is represented within the human body they developed a cosmology through the worship and scientific analysis of male and female bodies and deep introspective research into the secrets of birth, death, and immortality encoded in sex.

Tantra sexual practices are surrounded by ritual and practised in the context of meditation. The act of love between a man and a woman is sacred and held in the highest esteem, as an opportunity to embrace the most exalted spiritual states.

POSITIVE AND NEGATIVE POLES

Each of the first six Chakras (see page 251) are either receptive (Yin) or positive (Yang) poles. The male and female Chakra systems have opposite polarity except at the seventh Chakra, which is beyond duality. Between a man and a woman the opposite poles attract each other; imbalance at these poles can lead to problems in relating, either sexually or in day-to-day issues. The positive poles massage described in this chapter awakens and opens the Yang Chakras, and then the negative, Yin Chakras open automatically.

The male positive poles are the first, third, and fifth Chakras; the female positive poles are the second, fourth, and sixth Chakras. This massage focuses on each of the positive poles in turn, and then integrates this energy through the whole body, powerfully affecting the resonance between you.

When exchanging a massage with your lover, technique is not so important. What makes all the difference is loving, conscious touch. Focus on the touch you give, be present in it and enjoy it. Then your partner will also enjoy the massage, because a circle of giving and receiving is created between you, which will take you both into a space of deep and soul-nourishing intimacy.

Take turns to massage each other. Then you will be ready to enter into lovemaking from a place of heightened sensitivity and openness.

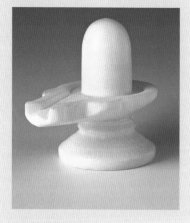

Yoni and Lingam
Tantra uses the Sanskrit names for the genitals, since these carry a profound message for enhancing pleasure. Lingam (the male genitals) means "pillar of light"; Yoni (the female genitals) means "sacred place". By transforming everyday sexuality into sacred sexuality, you lift the experience of sex into its refined aspect; it is a door leading to superconsciousness.

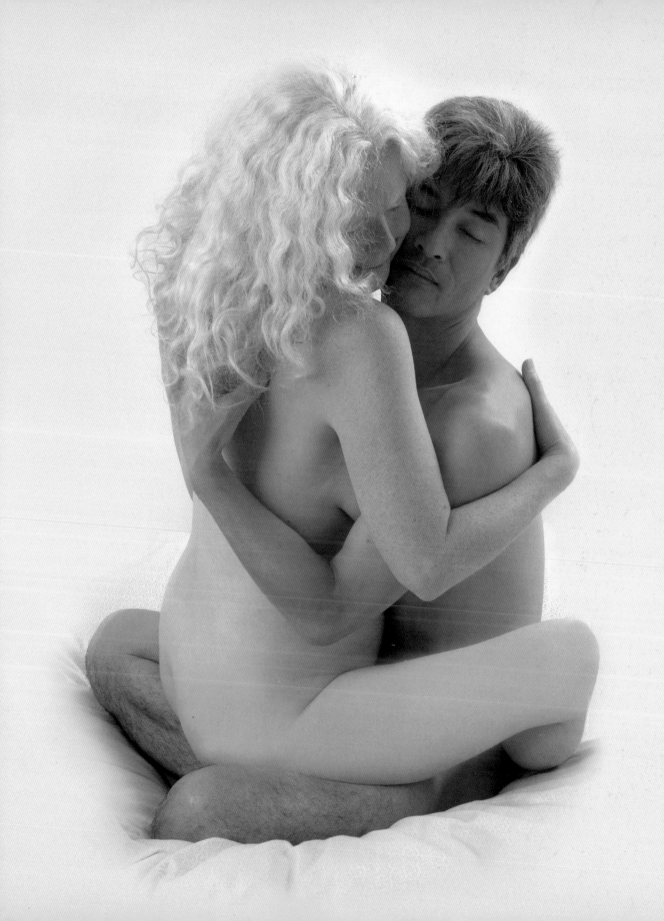

POSITIVE POLES MASSAGE

Step 1

Start on your partner's back, massaging all over the sacrum to awaken the energy in that area.

Step 2

Use your hands to move the energy that has been awakened in the sacrum by stroking up along either side of the spine. When you reach the top, move this energy through the shoulders and out through the arms and hands. Massaging the area in the centre of the back between the underarm folds will also free the energy flow in the genitals.

Step 3

Massage the back of the head lightly, then the backs of the legs and feet. Ask your partner to turn over and then start to massage the front of the legs and feet. Next focus on the inner thighs all the way up to the groin. Then follow the instructions for either the man (see facing page) or the woman (pages 238–9), as appropriate.

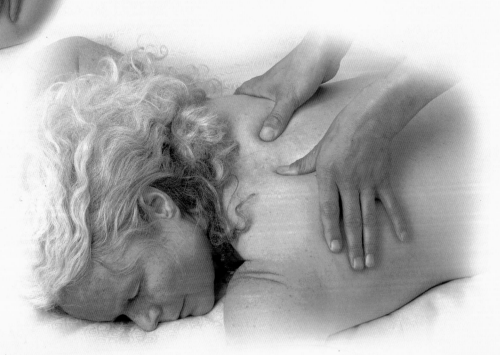

MASSAGE FOR THE MAN

Step 1
Massage the belly softly, making clockwise movements around the navel. Then focus on the solar plexus (third Chakra), between the ribcage and the navel. Complete the massage in this area by resting your relaxed hands for long moments on the solar plexus.

Step 2
Integrate the solar plexus energy into the rest of the body by stroking again around the whole belly and then stroking upward, letting your hands glide up and out along the shoulders, arms, and hands. Massage the arms and hands, and then come back to the neck and throat (fifth Chakra). Finish by resting one hand on the neck while the other rests lightly on the throat.

Step 3
Massage around the genitals at the groin and around where they are attached to the body (first Chakra). Then focus on the perineum point between the testicles and the anus.

Next massage the Lingam and testicles and cradle them in your hands. As you touch the Lingam, remember that the name means

"pillar of light". The emphasis is not on exciting your partner, but on loving, honouring, and relaxing tensions in that area.

Step 4
To complete the massage, integrate the energy from the genitals with the rest of the body by stroking down the legs and up the body, through the chest, across the

shoulders, and along the arms. Then rest your palms very lightly over the eyes for a few moments, allowing your partner to let go into a deeply nourishing silent space.

Finally lift your hands up and away from his body. Then Namaste to each other as a sign of gratitude (see page 239).

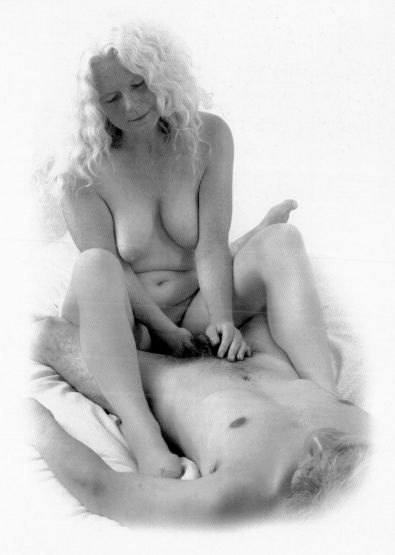

237

MASSAGE FOR THE WOMAN

Step 1

Massage the belly lightly and lovingly, with gentle movements, clockwise around the navel. Then rest your relaxed hands on the area between the pubic hair line and the navel (second Chakra) for a couple of minutes.

Step 2

Integrate the belly's energy with the rest of the body by stroking upward over the chest (fourth Chakra) and out along the arms and hands. Massage the breasts. (It may be helpful to ask the woman to show you how she likes to have her breasts massaged before you begin this massage.) As you massage her breasts, the emphasis is not on turning her on, but on honouring her as a goddess and drawing nourishment and love from them. Finish by stroking the awakened energy around the breasts and out through the arms and hands.

Step 3

Massage the arms and hands and then move up to the neck, scalp, and face. Stroke all over the neck, scalp, and ears and then the face. Focus on the forehead and between the eyebrows (sixth Chakra). Softly caress upward from the bridge of the nose to the hairline repeatedly for a couple of minutes, to open the third eye (seventh Chakra).

Step 4

Start massaging lightly around the Yoni and the groin area (first Chakra), then softly caress the Yoni and pubic hair, with great adoration and respect, remembering that Yoni means "sacred place". Use loving touch at the opening of the Yoni and on the clitoris. Your emphasis is not on arousing the woman, but on loving her.

Step 5

To complete the massage, integrate the energy from the genitals with the rest of the body by stroking down the legs and up the body, through the chest, across the shoulders, and along the arms. Then rest your relaxed hands on the belly, below the navel, for a few moments.

When you feel her sinking deeper into let go, you can slowly lift your hands off the body and hold them just above, allowing the second Chakra to expand even more. Lift your hands up and away from her body; then Namaste to each other as a sign of gratitude (see right).

Namaste

The Sanskrit word "Namaste" means "I bow down to the divine within you". Hold your hands together as for praying, in front of your chest, and look into your partner's eyes, as you bow slightly from the waist.

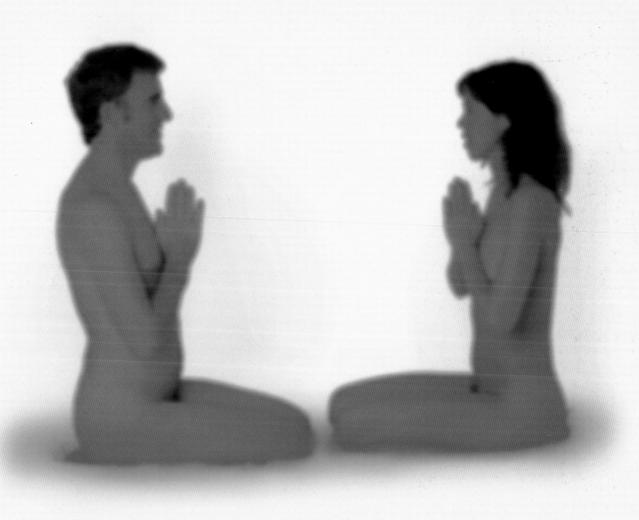

APPENDIX

THE CHANNELS

The illustrations show the course of each Channel (Meridian) on the surface of the body. All the Channels appear symmetrically on both sides of the body, except for the Ren and Du Channels which are on the midline.

Chinese massage and shiatsu both promote the smooth flow of life energy (known as Qi in Chinese massage, Ki in shiatsu) in the Channels.

Lung Channel

This Channel runs from the front of the shoulder, along the inside of the arm and ends at the corner of the thumbnail.

Large Intestine Channel

Starting at the tip of the index finger, this Channel passes through the back of the hand and up the back of the arm to the shoulder. It then curves above the collarbone and up the neck and cheek to end by the nostril.

Stomach Channel

This Channel begins just below the eye and curves round below the mouth, then back up over the cheek to the temple. From the jawbone it runs down the throat, along the collarbone, and then down the front of the body and leg to end at the tip of the second toe.

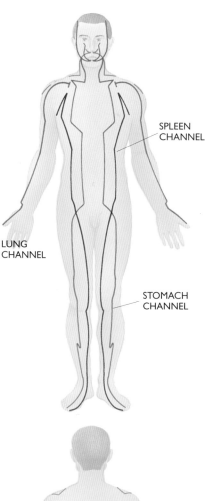

LUNG CHANNEL

SPLEEN CHANNEL

STOMACH CHANNEL

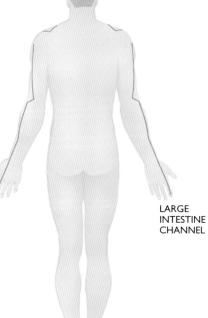

LARGE INTESTINE CHANNEL

Spleen Channel

The Spleen Channel begins at the tip of the big toe and climbs up the inside of the leg. It then runs up the abdomen to the chest, ending near the armpit.

Heart Channel

This Channel runs from the armpit down the inside of the arm, to end on the little finger.

Small Intestine Channel

Starting on the little finger, this Channel runs up the back of the arm, over the shoulder blade to the collarbone and up the cheek. There it divides, with one branch ending by the nose, the other by the ear.

Bladder Channel

From the inner corner of the eye, this Channel passes over the top of the head and branches at the nape to run down the back in two lines parallel to the spine. These two branches continue over the buttocks and down the back of the leg, reuniting at the knee. The Channel ends at the tip of the little toe.

Kidney Channel

This Channel starts at the little toe and passes along the sole of the foot before proceeding up the inside of the leg to the top of the inner thigh. From here it passes up the side of the abdomen and finishes near the armpit.

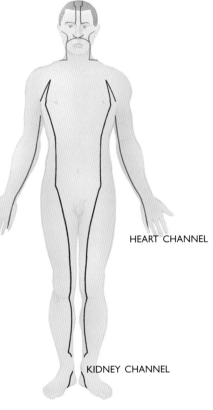

HEART CHANNEL

KIDNEY CHANNEL

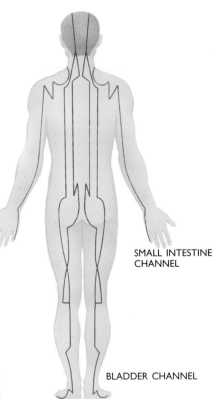

SMALL INTESTINE
CHANNEL

BLADDER CHANNEL

Pericardium Channel

In Oriental medicine, the Pericardium is sometimes known as the Heart Protector. It has no equivalent in Western medicine. This Channel starts above the nipple and flows down the arm to end at the tip of the middle finger.

Triple Warmer Channel

The Triple Warmer has no equivalent in Western medicine. In Oriental medicine it is the passageway for Qi (or Ki) and fluids through the abdomen, but it has no physical counterpart. The Channel starts at the tip of the fourth finger and runs up the back of the arm to the shoulder, up the neck, and over the top of the ear to end at the outer edge of the eye.

Gall Bladder Channel

This Channel starts at the outer edge of the eye socket and winds over the head, down to the nape of the head. It then zigzags down the side of the body and continues down the outside of the leg to end at the tip of the fourth toe.

Liver Channel

Starting at the big toe, this Channel passes over the top of the foot and ascends the inside of the leg to the groin, then up the sides of the abdomen to end on the chest.

Ren and Du Channels

In Oriental medicine these are known as "extra Channels" and they are not associated with an organ of the body. The Ren Channel runs up the midline from the perineum to the lower lip. The Du Channel runs up from the upper lip over the back of the head and down the spine, ending at the perineum.

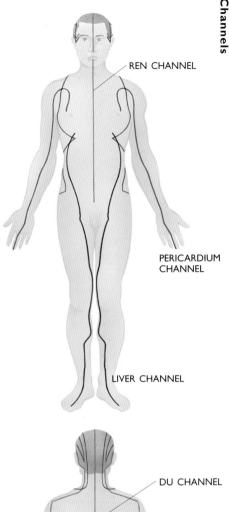

REN CHANNEL

PERICARDIUM
CHANNEL

LIVER CHANNEL

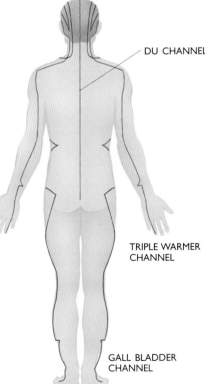

DU CHANNEL

TRIPLE WARMER
CHANNEL

GALL BLADDER
CHANNEL

THE ACUPOINTS

The diagrams show the position of the most commonly used acupoints. The descriptions explain in more detail how to locate the acupoints used in this book (see page 252 for body landmark diagrams). Remember that all acupoints appear symmetrically on both sides of the body, except for those on the Ren and Du Channels.

BACK

B12 4 cm (1.5 in) either side of the spine, level with the 2nd thoracic vertebra.

B13 4 cm (1.5 in) either side of the spine, level with the 3rd thoracic vertebra.

B15 4 cm (1.5 in) either side of the spine, level with the 5th thoracic vertebra.

B18 4 cm (1.5 in) either side of the spine, level with the 9th thoracic vertebra.

B19 4 cm (1.5 in) either side of the spine, level with the 10th thoracic vertebra.

B20 4 cm (1.5 in) either side of the spine, level with the 11th thoracic vertebra.

B21 4 cm (1.5 in) either side of the spine, level with the12th thoracic vertebra.

B23 4 cm (1.5 in) either side of the spine, level with the 2nd lumbar vertebra.

B25 4 cm (1.5 in) either side of the spine, level with the 4th lumbar vertebra.

B27 4 cm (1.5 in) either side of the spine, level with the 1st sacral foramina.

B31–B34 4 cm (1.5 in) either side of the spine, on the sacrum.

Du14 On the back of the neck between the 7th cervical and 1st

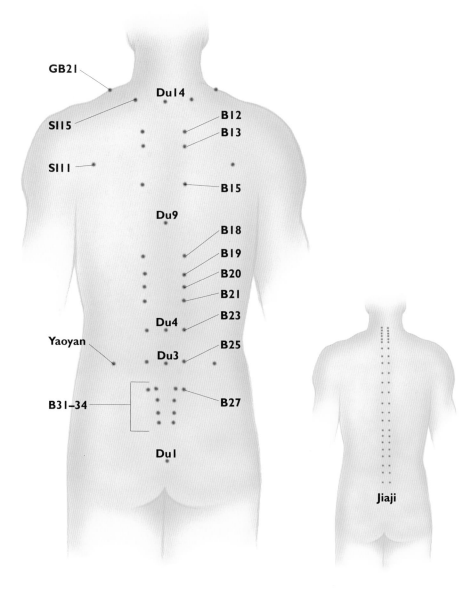

thoracic vertebrae. The 7th cervical is the prominent bone on the back of the neck when the head is bent forward.

GB21 In the middle of the top of the shoulder, midway between the 7th cervical vertebra and the outermost edge of the shoulder blade.

Jiaji Extra points 1 cm (0.5 in) either side of the spine, from the neck to the lumbar region.

SI11 The midpoint of the shoulder blade.

SI15 5 cm (2 in) either side of the midline of the back, level with the 7th cervical and 1st thoracic vertebrae.

Yaoyan About 10 cm (4 in) either side of the spine, level with the 4th lumbar vertebra.

ARM AND HAND

H7 On the little finger end of the wrist crease.

LI1 On the corner of the index fingernail nearest the thumb.

LI10 5 cm (2 in) down from the thumb side of the elbow crease.

LI11 On the thumb side of the elbow crease, found when the arm is bent.

LI15 In the dimple 5 cm (2 in) below the outer edge of the shoulder, found when the arm is raised sideways.

LI4 On the back of the hand, in the web between the thumb and index finger.

LI5 In the hollow in the wrist, just off the base of the thumb, found when the thumb points upward.

Lu10 4 cm (1.5 in) from the wrist crease, along the palm side of the thumb.

Lu11 On the outside corner of the thumbnail bed.

Lu5 On the outside of the elbow crease, found when the arm is slightly bent.

Lu7 4 cm (1.5 in) above the wrist crease, on the thumb side of the inner forearm.

Lu9 In the depression on the thumb side of the wrist crease.

P3 At the elbow crease, on the inside of the biceps tendon, found when the arm is slightly bent.

P6 5 cm (2 in) from the wrist crease, in the middle of the inner forearm.

P8 In the middle of the palm.

P9 At the tip of the middle finger.

SI1 On the outside corner of the little fingernail.

SI3 At the end of the palm crease, on the little finger side of the hand, found when the fist is slightly clenched.

SI8 In the depression in the back of the elbow, found when the arm is bent.

SI9 2.5 cm (1 in) above the end of the posterior armpit crease.

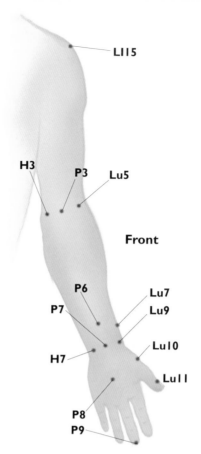
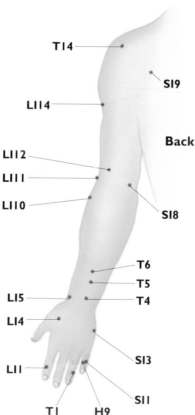

T1 On the corner of the 4th fingernail, on the little finger side.

T14 In the dimple below the edge of the shoulder on the back of the body, about 2.5 cm (1 in) behind LI15.

T4 In the dimple in the middle of the wrist on the back of the hand.

T5 5 cm (2 in) above the midpoint of the wrist on the back of the hand.

T6 7.5 cm (3 in) above the midpoint of the wrist on the back of the forearm.

Channel abbreviations

The acupoints are labelled according to the Channel on which they lie, using the following abbreviations:

Lu *Lung Channel*
LI *Large Intestine Channel*
St *Stomach Channel*
H *Heart Channel*
SI *Small Intestine Channel*
B *Bladder Channel*
K *Kidney Channel*
P *Pericardium Channel*
T *Triple Warmer Channel*
GB *Gall Bladder Channel*
Liv *Liver Channel*
Du *Du Channel*
Ren *Ren Channel*

Some extra points do not lie on the Channels, and are known by name only, for example "Heding".

ABDOMEN

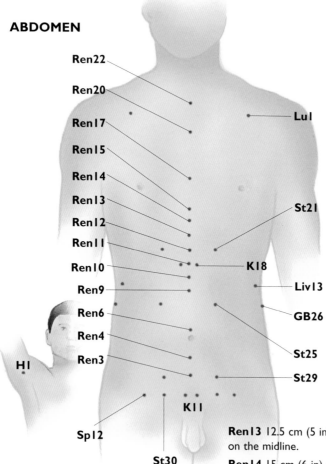

Ren22
Ren20
Ren17
Ren15
Ren14
Ren13
Ren12
Ren11
Ren10
Ren9
Ren6
Ren4
Ren3

Lu1
St21
K18
Liv13
GB26
St25
St29

H1

K11

Sp12
St30

HEAD

B2 On the inner end of the eyebrow.

Du16 In the hollow under the protuberance on the midline, just above the hairline on the back of the head.

Du20 On the top of the head, midway between the ears.

Du23 Two finger widths above the forehead hairline, on the midline.

GB20 At the base of the skull in the hollow in the hairline, between the front and back neck muscles behind the bony prominence behind the ear.

GB8 Two finger widths directly above the top of the ear.

LI20 At the base of the nose, either side of the nostrils.

SI19 Between the jaw joint and the front of the ear, in the depression formed when the mouth opens.

St1 Directly below the pupil, on the lower edge of the eye socket.

St2 In the depression roughly 2.5 cm (1 in) directly below the pupil.

St21 10 cm (4 in) above the navel and 5 cm (2 in) either side of the midline of the belly.

St25 5 cm (2 in) either side of the navel.

St29 10 cm (4 in) below the navel and 5 cm (2 in) either side of the midline of the belly.

St30 12.5 cm (5 in) below the navel and 5 cm (2 in) either side of the midline of the belly.

St6 2.5 cm (1 in) diagonally up from the corner of the lower jaw.

St7 In the depression about 2.5 cm (1 in) in front of the ear, found when the mouth shuts.

St8 Just inside the hairline at the corner of the forehead.

Taiyang On the temples, about 2.5 cm (1 in) beyond the eye socket, on a line from the eye to the top of the ear.

Yintang Just above the nose, between the eyebrows.

GB26 On the side of the abdomen, directly below the armpit and level with the navel.

H1 On the midpoint of the armpit.

K11 13 cm (5 in) below the navel, on the midline of the belly.

K18 7 cm (3 in) above the navel, 1 cm (0.5 in) either side of the midline.

Liv13 Stand with your arms hanging down by your sides and mark the points that your elbows reach.

Lu1 2.5 cm (1 in) below the collar bone at the shoulder end, and 15 cm (6 in) either side of the midline.

Ren10 5 cm (2 in) above the navel, on the midline.

Ren11 7.5 cm (3 in) above the navel, on the midline.

Ren12 10 cm (4 in) above the navel, on the midline.

Ren13 12.5 cm (5 in) above the navel, on the midline.

Ren14 15 cm (6 in) above the navel, on the midline.

Ren15 1 cm (0.5 in) below the breastbone, on the midline.

Ren17 On the breastbone, midway between the nipples.

Ren20 7.5 cm (3 in) directly below the top of the breastbone, on the midline.

Ren22 In the hollow 1 cm (0.5 in) above the top of the breastbone, on the midline.

Ren3 10 cm (4 in) below the navel, on the midline.

Ren4 7.5 cm (3 in) below the navel, on the midline.

Ren6 4 cm (1.5 in) below the navel, on the midline.

Ren9 2.5 cm (1 in) above the navel, on the midline.

Sp12 9 cm (3.5 in) either side of the midline, on the same level as the top of the pubic bone.

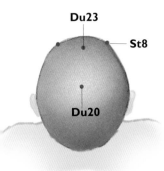

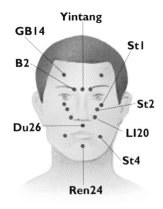

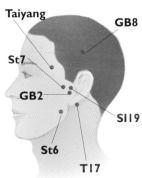

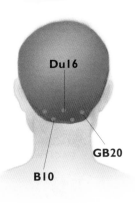

FOOT AND LEG

B36 In the midpoint of the crease below the buttock.

B37 15 cm (6 in) below the crease of the buttock, in the middle of the back of the leg.

B40 In the midpoint of the knee crease on the back of the leg.

B57 In the middle of the back of the calf, midway between the knee crease and the heel.

B60 On the outside of the ankle joint, midway between the ankle bone and the Achilles tendon.

GB30 On the side of the buttocks, two thirds of the way toward the top of the thigh bone from the sacrum.

GB31 Standing with your arms relaxed, the tip of your middle finger reaches this point on the outside of your thigh.

GB34 On the outside of the lower leg in a depression just in front of and a little below the head of the fibula.

GB39 7.5 cm (3 in) above the ankle bone on the outside of the lower leg.

GB40 In the depression diagonally below the outside ankle bone.

Heding The depression on the upper edge of the kneecap, found when the leg is bent.

K1 On the midline of the sole of the foot, at the colour change between ball and sole.

K3 Midway between the inside ankle joint and the Achilles tendon.

K6 In the depression one thumb width below the inside ankle bone.

Liv8 On the inner end of the crease at the back of the knee.

Liv3 On the top of the foot, in the furrow between the 1st and 2nd toes, where the bones merge.

Sp10 5 cm (2 in) above the top of the kneecap, in line with its inside edge.

Sp4 On the inside arch of the foot, about 2.5 cm (1 in) behind the long bone of the big toe.

Sp6 7.5 cm (3 in) above the inside ankle joint.

Sp9 Below the knee joint, in the depression between the tibia and the calf muscle, on the inside lower leg.

St31 On the line between the kneecap and the pelvic bone, level with the genital region.

St32 15 cm (6 in) above the top of the kneecap, in line with its outside edge.

St34 5 cm (2 in) above the top of the kneecap, in line with its outside edge.

St36 7.5 cm (3 in) below the kneecap, on the outside of the leg.

St40 20 cm (8 in) above the outside ankle joint.

St41 In the depression in the middle of the front of the ankle joint, between the tendons.

Xiyan In the two depressions of the knee joint, just below the kneecap, found when the knee is bent.

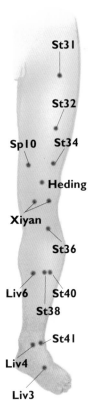

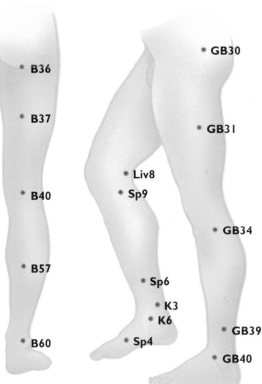

REFLEXOLOGY – FEET

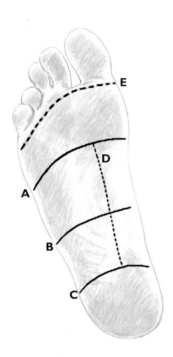

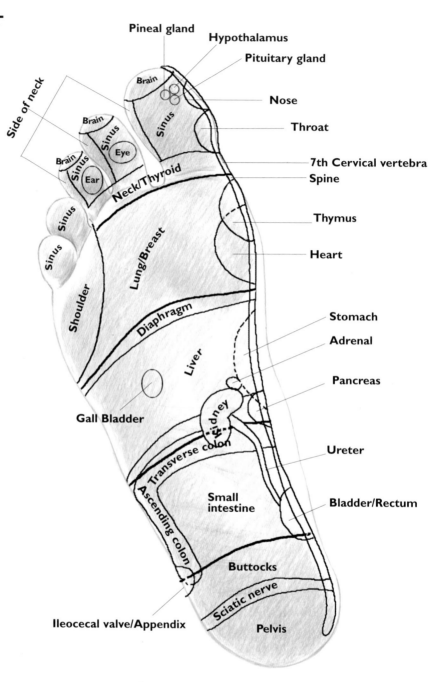

The diaphragm line (A), the waist line (B), the pelvic line (C) and the ligament line (D) divide the feet into sections relating to areas of the body. The shoulder line is a secondary guideline.

Reflexes relating to the heart and lungs lie above the diaphragm line. Reflexes for the digestive system, kidneys, and spleen lie between the waist and diaphragm lines. Reflexes for the organs of elimination lie between the pelvic and waist lines. Reflexes for the reproductive organs lie below the pelvic line. Reflexes for the sinuses, eyes, ears, thyroid, and neck lie above the shoulder line.

Use the maps on this and the following pages to help you locate all the reflexes on the hands and feet. Each area mapped contains many reflex points, rather like pins on a pincushion, but they are referred to as the heart reflex, stomach reflex, etc. The areas overlap, so when you work one area you will often contact reflex points in another.

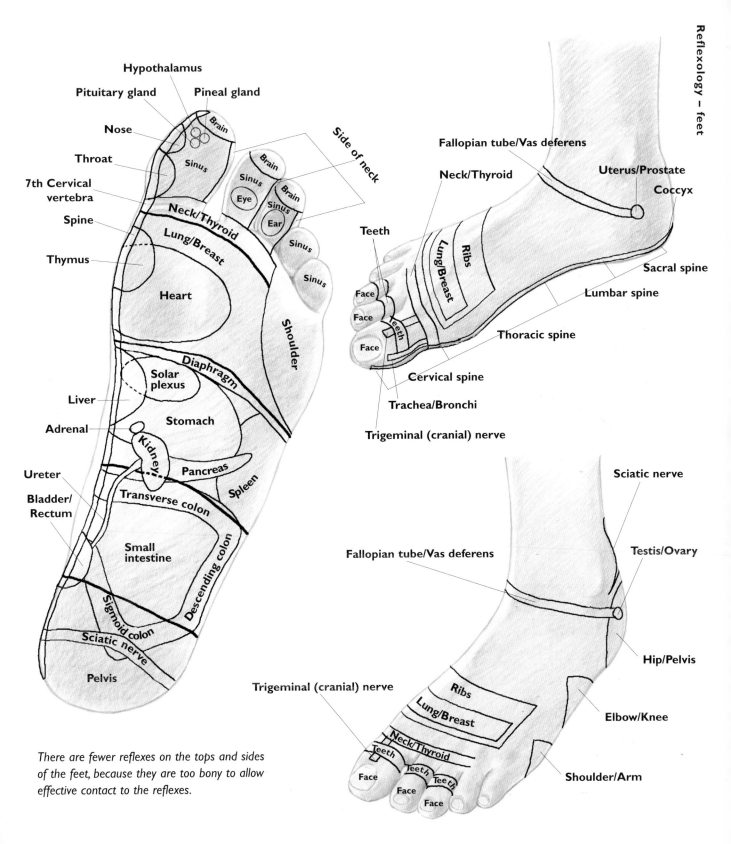

Hypothalamus
Pituitary gland
Pineal gland
Nose
Throat
7th Cervical vertebra
Spine
Thymus
Side of neck
Brain
Sinus
Brain
Sinus
Eye
Brain
Sinus
Ear
Sinus
Sinus
Neck/Thyroid
Lung/Breast
Heart
Shoulder
Diaphragm
Solar plexus
Liver
Stomach
Adrenal
Kidney
Pancreas
Spleen
Ureter
Bladder/Rectum
Transverse colon
Small intestine
Descending colon
Sigmoid colon
Sciatic nerve
Pelvis

Fallopian tube/Vas deferens
Neck/Thyroid
Uterus/Prostate
Coccyx
Teeth
Lung/Breast
Ribs
Face
Face
Teeth
Face
Sacral spine
Lumbar spine
Thoracic spine
Cervical spine
Trachea/Bronchi
Trigeminal (cranial) nerve

Sciatic nerve
Fallopian tube/Vas deferens
Testis/Ovary
Hip/Pelvis
Elbow/Knee
Trigeminal (cranial) nerve
Ribs
Lung/Breast
Neck/Thyroid
Teeth
Face
Teeth
Teeth
Face
Face
Shoulder/Arm

There are fewer reflexes on the tops and sides of the feet, because they are too bony to allow effective contact to the reflexes.

REFLEXOLOGY – HANDS

The hands are smaller, which means that the hand reflexes are condensed and much less obvious than those on the feet.

Right hand

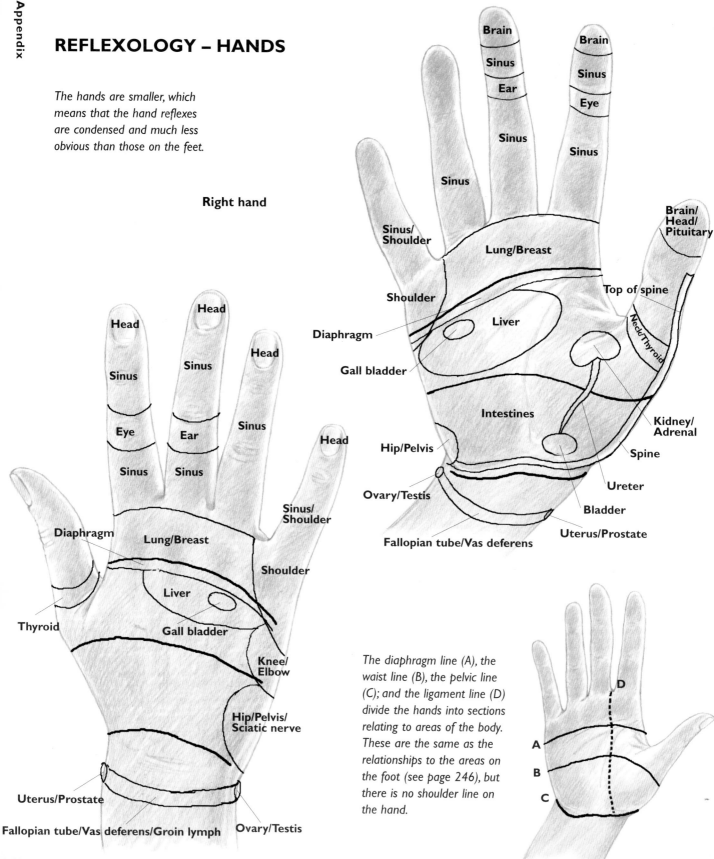

The diaphragm line (A), the waist line (B), the pelvic line (C); and the ligament line (D) divide the hands into sections relating to areas of the body. These are the same as the relationships to the areas on the foot (see page 246), but there is no shoulder line on the hand.

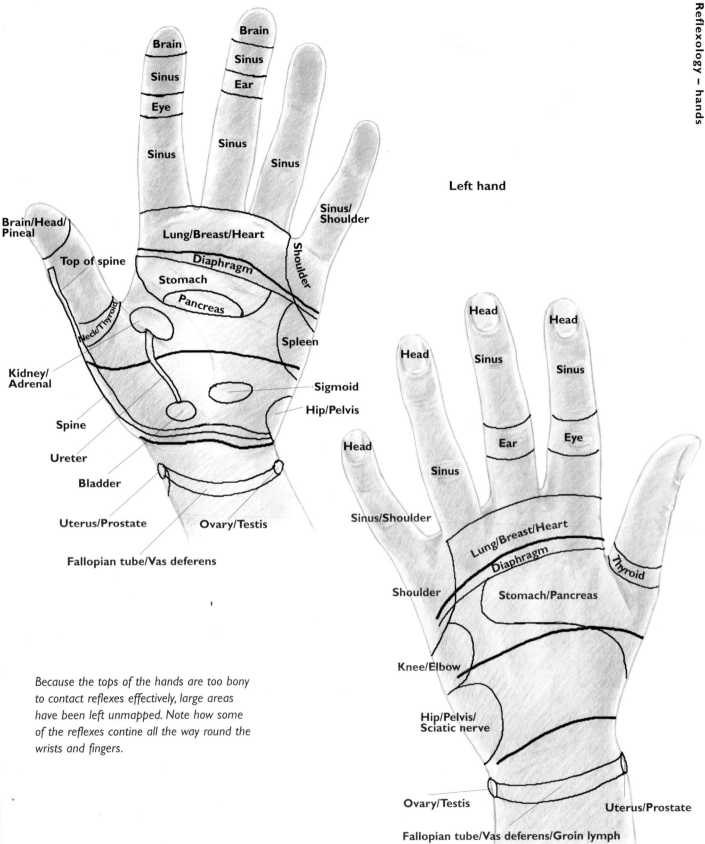

Brain
Sinus
Eye
Sinus

Brain
Sinus
Ear
Sinus

Sinus

Sinus/Shoulder

Left hand

Brain/Head/Pineal

Top of spine

Lung/Breast/Heart

Diaphragm

Shoulder

Stomach

Pancreas

Neck/Thyroid

Spleen

Kidney/Adrenal

Spine

Sigmoid

Hip/Pelvis

Ureter

Bladder

Uterus/Prostate

Ovary/Testis

Fallopian tube/Vas deferens

Head

Head

Head

Sinus

Sinus

Head

Sinus

Ear

Eye

Sinus/Shoulder

Lung/Breast/Heart

Diaphragm

Thyroid

Shoulder

Stomach/Pancreas

Knee/Elbow

Hip/Pelvis/Sciatic nerve

Ovary/Testis

Uterus/Prostate

Fallopian tube/Vas deferens/Groin lymph

Because the tops of the hands are too bony to contact reflexes effectively, large areas have been left unmapped. Note how some of the reflexes contine all the way round the wrists and fingers.

249

AROMATHERAPY OILS

OIL	QUALITIES
Benzoin	soothe, stabilize, nurture
Bergamot[1]	release, relax, uplift
Caraway[2]	steadfast determination, confident commitment
Cardamom	appetite, stability, contentment
Cedarwood	strength, endurance, certainty
Chamomile	calm control, easy acceptance
Clary Sage[4]	revitalize, clarify, inspire
Coriander	joyful stability, calm creativity
Eucalyptus[5]	optimism, openness, freedom
Frankincense	tranquil contemplation, spiritual liberation
Geranium	security, receptivity, intimacy
Ginger	initiative, self-confidence, accomplishment
Jasmine	desire, creativity, harmony
Juniper[4,5]	fortify, unburden, empower
Lavender	calm composure, easy self-expression
Lemon[3]	refreshing, clear, trusting
Marjoram[4]	comfort, contentment, compassion
Myrrh	tranquil solitude, transcendent peace
Neroli	reassurance, retrieval, renewal
Orange	ease, adaptability, optimism
Palmarosa	secure, fluid, adaptable
Patchouli	earthing, arousing, enriching
Peppermint[4]	attentive, tolerant, visionary
Pine	distinct self-identity, vibrant self-image
Rose	love, trust, self-acceptance
Rosemary[4]	self-identity, dedication, destiny
Sandalwood	stillness, unity, being
Tea tree	strength, resistance, confidence
Vetiver	nourishing, restoring, reconnecting
Yarrow[4]	protecting, mollifying, healing
Ylang Ylang	relaxing, sensualizing, euphoric

Safety notes

1 Avoid exposure to direct sunlight for 12 hours after application.

2 Mild irritant of mucous membranes.

3 Avoid exposure to direct sunlight for 4 hours after application.

4 Do not use in pregnancy or while breast-feeding, or on children under two years. Avoid using on individuals with epilepsy, fever, or heart disease. Do not use at more than 2% dilution or more than 1 ml per 24 hours (adult).

5 Do not use on anyone with kidney problems.

THE CHAKRAS

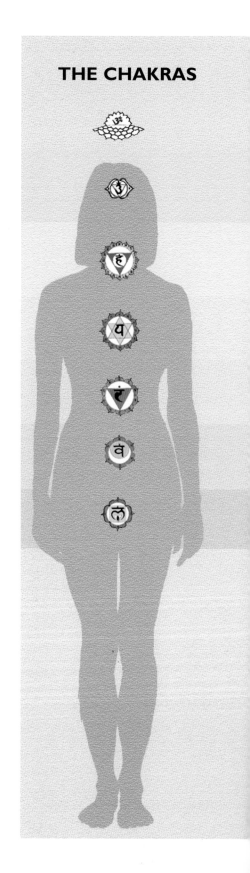

NAME	ORGAN	THEME
Crown (Seventh) Chakra	Upper brain, right eye, pineal gland	Consciousness of oneness, spiritual awareness, extended consciousness, wisdom, intuition, connection to the Higher Self, to the inner guidance, and to all-embracing love
Third eye (Sixth) Chakra	Lower brain, left eye, nose, spine, ears, pituitary gland	Clairvoyance, telepathy, seat of will, thought control, inner vision and understanding, inspiration, spiritual awakening
Throat (Fifth) Chakra	Throat, thyroid gland, upper lung and arms, digestive tract	Self expression, communication, creativity, sense of responsibility
Heart (Fourth) Chakra	Heart, lungs, circulation, thymus gland	Centre of the emotions, love for self and others, peace, sympathy, forgiveness, trust, spiritual development, compassion
Solar Plexus (Third) Chakra	Stomach, liver, gall bladder, pancreas, solar plexus	Power, dominance, strength, fear
Sacral (Second) Chakra	Reproductive organs, urogenital system, kidneys, gonads, legs	Vitality, enjoyment of life, self-esteem, refinement of feelings, relationships, desire
Root (First) Chakra	Adrenal glands, bladder, genitals, spine	Will to live, life force, survival, fertility, procreation

BODY LANDMARKS

Use these illustrations to help you identify the main bones and anatomical features that are used as body landmarks for locating acupoints and in the massage sequences.

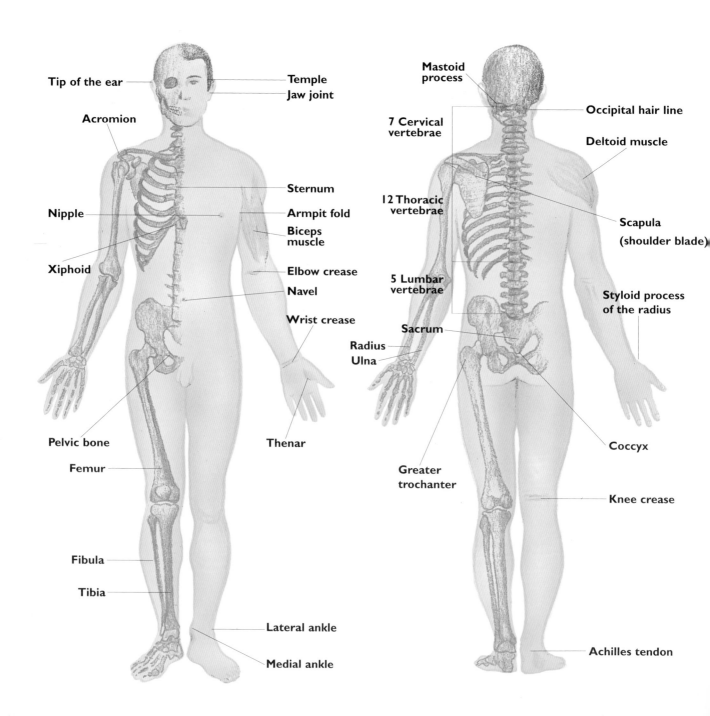

Tip of the ear
Temple
Jaw joint
Acromion
Sternum
Nipple
Armpit fold
Biceps muscle
Xiphoid
Elbow crease
Navel
Wrist crease
Pelvic bone
Thenar
Femur
Fibula
Tibia
Lateral ankle
Medial ankle

Mastoid process
Occipital hair line
7 Cervical vertebrae
Deltoid muscle
12 Thoracic vertebrae
Scapula (shoulder blade)
5 Lumbar vertebrae
Styloid process of the radius
Sacrum
Radius
Ulna
Coccyx
Greater trochanter
Knee crease
Achilles tendon

INDEX

ACKNOWLEDGEMENTS

The publisher would like to
thank: Sheilagh Noble for new
illustrations; Kasia Posen and
Catherine Walpole for
modelling for photographs;
Camilla Davis and Deborah
Pate for typing; Jane Parker
for the index.

Gaia Books would like to
acknowledge the use of text
from the following books (all
published by Gaia Books):
*Acupressure for Common
Ailments*, Chris Jarmey and
John Tindall
*A Gaia Busy Person's Guide:
Massage*, Eilean Bentley
*A Gaia Busy Person's Guide:
Reflexology*, Ann Gillanders
*Aromatherapy for Common
Ailments*, Shirley Price
*Aromatherapy for Healing the
Spirit*, Gabriel Mojay
Inner Reiki, Tanmaya
Honervogt
*Reflexology: A Step by Step
Guide*, Ann Gillanders
*Reiki: Healing and Harmony
Through the Hands*, Tanmaya
Honervogt
Step by Step Head Massage,
Eilean Bentley
*Step by Step Massage for Pain
Relief*, Peijian Shen
Tantric Sex, Ma Ananda Sarita
and Swami Anand Geho
The New Book of Massage,
Lucy Lidell
The New Book of Shiatsu, Paul
Lundberg